Breaking Through to Teens

"*Breaking Through to Teens* is a book that has value as both a comprehensive first read and as a text used for frequent, repeated reference in work with young adults....Leaving this text is like leaving a good professional workshop or conference. You are inspired, reminded of old concepts, enlightened by old concepts in new frames, and interested in learning more about new concepts just introduced. You have smiled and grinned, been challenged to think, and perhaps even made a new friend. Social workers, psychologists, parents, and those whose work gives them the honor of interacting with adolescents all stand to gain from this inspiring new approach to our new adolescents." —*Child and Adolescent Social Work Journal*

"This is a remarkable book written by a renowned psychologist and therapist. Dr. Taffel presents a new, exciting approach for working with adolescents of the 21st century. He describes this approach with exquisite clarity and vivid case examples, and in the process challenges long-held views of existing therapy models. Every page bears witness to Dr. Taffel's empathy and warmth and his understanding of adolescents and their families. This book is a wonderful resource for both beginning and experienced therapists, and should also serve as a major text in courses in counseling and therapy."—**Robert Brooks, PhD, Harvard Medical School**

"Dr. Taffel returns from the front lines of working with kids and parents, with scary yet hopeful stories of what he sees today. His account is bold, honest, and clear. What we used to call 'at-risk' behavior is now normal teen behavior. America faces an epidemic of culturally induced anxiety in teens. Parents are not really in control. For clinicians who feel in over their heads with today's teens and families (and who doesn't?), thanks to this book, help is on the way." —**Mary Pipher, PhD, author of** *Reviving Ophelia*

"From the numerous, specific case examples and therapy dialogues, to precise questions to consider and ask, this book fills a hunger that therapists—like the parents and adolescents they treat—have for guidance without equivocation. Graduate students, beginning clinicians, and experienced practitioners will find here a powerful approach to making and sustaining transformative alliances with these most challenging cases." —**Martha B. Straus, PhD, Department of Clinical Psychology, Antioch New England Graduate School**

"In this radical and exciting book, Dr. Taffel issues a challenge to counselors and therapists working with teenagers: Stop being so passive! Rethink the old rules! In this shrink-savvy generation, kids are expert at manipulating their parents and their therapists. Dr. Taffel offers many specific, helpful suggestions for getting teens into therapy and for getting them to stop their self-destructive behaviors." —**Michael Thompson, PhD, coauthor of** *Raising Cain*

"An excellent resource for professionals working with teens or their parents."—*Youth Today*

BREAKING THROUGH TO TEENS

Psychotherapy for the New Adolescence

RON TAFFEL

THE GUILFORD PRESS
New York / London

© 2005 The Guilford Press
A Division of Guilford Publications, Inc.
72 Spring Street, New York, NY 10012
www.guilford.com

Paperback edition 2010

Printed in the United States of America

This book is printed on acid-free paper.

Last digit is print number: 9 8 7 6 5 4 3

Library of Congress Cataloging-in-Publication Data

Taffel, Ron.
    Breaking through to teens : psychotherapy for the new
adolescence / Ron Taffel.
        p.; cm.
    Includes bibliographical references and index.
    ISBN 978-1-59385-135-4 (hardcover: alk. paper)
    ISBN 978-1-60623-944-5 (paperback: alk. paper)
    1. Adolescent psychotherapy.   2. Parent and teenager.
    [DNLM: 1. Psychotherapy—methods—Adolescent.
    2. Adolescent Psychology.   3. Parent–Child Relations.
    4. Professional–Patient Relations.   WS 463 T124b 2005]
    I. Title.
    RJ503.T34 2005
    616.89′00835—dc22

                                                    2004027861

The hardcover edition of *Breaking Through to Teens*
(ISBN 978-1-59385-135-4) has the subtitle
"A New Psychotherapy for the New Adolescence."

*To Leah and Sam, our teens at home—
and to all the kids in these pages:
Snowflakes on a winter's wind that
brought them into the springtime
of their lives*

ABOUT THE AUTHOR

Ron Taffel, PhD, has supervised and written about working with children and families for over two decades. He is one of the country's most sought-after speakers for both professional and parent audiences. Dr. Taffel is the award-winning author of over 100 academic and popular articles, and has been a contributing editor to *McCall's* and *Parents* magazines for 14 years. His childrearing guides, translated into numerous languages, include the critically acclaimed *Parenting by Heart, Nurturing Good Children Now, When Parents Disagree,* and *The Second Family,* as well as the professional handbooks *Getting Through to Difficult Kids and Parents* and *Breaking Through to Teens.* Dr. Taffel is the founder of Family and Couples Treatment Services at The Institute for Contemporary Psychotherapy in New York City, where he lives with his wife and two children.

ACKNOWLEDGMENTS

Adolescents have parents who affect them in obvious ways. They also have peer groups or, as I call them, "second families"—that profoundly affect them in mostly invisible ways. Throughout this book, I openly acknowledge my professional "parents." I take great pains to mention almost every supervisor and writer who influenced me during my career. I have had the good fortune of being able to synthesize the material they offered and to use it as patients' needs and the context changed. Without sophisticated input from all of the sources you will find attributed in these pages, this work couldn't, wouldn't, and shouldn't have happened.

Like a teen's second family, however, several peer-group influences do not appear in this text and deserve to be mentioned. First, The Guilford Press. I have had good experiences with other publishers, and yet rarely have I found the degree of collaboration that exists at Guilford, and in unexpected ways: Like everything else of far greater importance, the writing of this book was set back after September 11, 2001. Most of you do not realize that The Guilford Press is situated quite close to the site of the attacks—they, like all of us, were profoundly affected by that horrific event. The people at Guilford were kind to me, a strange word to use in business, but they were. They never pushed me to ignore the clinical and service commitments I needed to fulfill as our city recovered. I can't thank them enough for this. For their unselfish grasp of what was truly important, I am forever indebted to Seymour Weingarten, Editor-in-Chief, and Bob Matloff, President, of The Guilford Press.

In terms of the book itself, it is rare to experience vision, practicality, and clinical sense from an editor—a combination I felt continuously from another invisible peer, Kathryn Moore, Executive Editor at Guilford. Kathryn is one of the most clinically astute and market-savvy editors I know. It is easy working with her because of these gifts, and also because she succeeds at creating what we therapists try to create: an ability to speak openly and then seriously work through difficult issues. Other authors in the field: If you have a chance to work with Kathryn, jump at it.

In addition, a book is not just a book. It is an organization, which is really a collection of peers who try very hard to do the best they can. Paul Gordon designed the cover, Kim Miller was responsible for pre-publicity, Katherine Lieber wrote the promotional copy, Jeanne Ford worked at copyediting, Anna Brackett did the interior book design and production, Sarah Smith provided creative input—all within a ridiculous timetable. Real people always exist behind the scenes in organizations; we just don't see them. But, without such peers, we literally wouldn't have books to read.

The second organization represented in the text is my professional peer group, The Institute for Contemporary Psychotherapy (ICP). In 1982 ICP had the foresight to grant the family therapy division I founded full political and curriculum parity in one of New York's most respected psychoanalytic training and treatment facilities. Their prescience was unique, as only now training facilities are finally attempting to lessen the distance between treatment perspectives rather than accentuate them. ICP has a history of such prescience and the courage to take initiative before an area of need is recognized: In the '70s they began The Center for the Study of Anorexia and Bulimia, the first eating disorders program in the country; at the same time ICP began one of the first low-fee programs for children, college students, and performing and creative artists; in the '80s ICP was one of the first independent facilities to treat HIV and AIDS patients and open its treatment doors to the elderly; in the mid-'90s ICP began one of the first and perhaps most successful gay and lesbian affirmative psychotherapy programs in the country; after 9/11 ICP threw hundreds of therapists into volunteer work with a generosity that was startling; and it has continued its commitment to treating trauma clients and educating professionals in the newest interventions. This is an organization that obviously has clinical foresight and determination, training thousands of professionals and treating 25,000 clients over three decades. I could not have developed the form of therapy described in these pages without the full support of ICP, and without my peer and original training director, Judith Friedman.

Finally, I would like to acknowledge *Psychotherapy Networker* and Rich Simon, its Editor-in-Chief. Again, in the background, another peer group quietly working: The entire organization and, of course, Rich gave me a platform for the approach outlined in this book. Look through my *Networker* articles over the past decade and you will see threads of the material taking shape and gradually being woven together. How can you thank colleagues enough when they've actually helped you to develop your own voice?

Adults, not just teens, have peer groups, which are more sustaining than we realize. The organizations I mention here have been my "second family" of peers, who strengthened me as I've developed and invisibly helped write the words on these pages, while granting me the independence to grow in my own unique ways.

CONTENTS

INTRODUCTION

A New World

I am repeatedly stunned when I am told that kids are no different today than they were when we were growing up. The underlying assumption is that we need not do anything differently
with our teen clients now than when we were first trained. Yet
how can it be that everything in the world has changed so significantly over the past few decades and somehow kids remain
the same? This notion has disastrous consequences. Adolescents
don't feel understood by adults, even by many professionals.
Adults don't know how to break through to kids. Parents feel
overwhelmed by ordinary teen life. Teens make decisions that put
them in harm's way.

In a crunch, families turn to child professionals, who often
don't know how to sort out the maze of contradictory childrearing
advice and therapeutic interventions, or who don't know how to
match treatment with a teen world that has dramatically shifted—
along with values about race, gender, family, marriage and divorce,
tradition, technology, and how kids define sex, abstinence, and
drinking. There is no way for us to help teenagers and their parents
unless we reexamine the way we work, so that we do not recreate
the parallel disconnection that exists in the homes we are supposed to help.

My Hopes

It is risky to go out on a limb and state exactly what one would like a book to accomplish. But working with kids is inspiring. Our two feisty adolescents at home remind us every day how nothing is accomplished without putting oneself on the line. Kids teach us to take risks with our spirit, with our intellect, and with our hearts. So, here are some of my hopes.

Most important, and without a moment's hesitation, I hope this book saves lives. I hope it will be a contribution that empowers our therapeutic efforts, work that is humbling to anyone willing to give it a try. I hope that you will find coherence in this model, that you will feel spoken to directly, and that your dilemmas with teenagers will be understood. I hope you will experience me to be a supportive but challenging voice that encourages you to think creatively and fight the alternating exhilaration and disappointment that comes with this territory. And, I hope that any confusion you feel from the endless stream of pop culture in combination with theoretical background noise begins to adhere into a coherent perspective that fits kids' lives today.

That's a lot to hope for. But adolescence is about just this kind of audacious yearning. One can't possibly work with teens without some of their spirit moving us in unexpected ways.

Toward a Measure of Coherence

Parents and child professionals are in a surprisingly similar predicament. We are inundated with new techniques and information that changes weekly about how to handle what I call "the new adolescence." The confusion of clinicians is apparent at every professional seminar I give, just as it is with every parent group I speak to. The model in this book is for everyone who has ever felt at sea with 21st century adolescents—which I believe is most of us, much of the time. It is aimed at the widest range of teens and parents possible. A word of caution: the approach is not geared for actively suicidal or program-worthy substance-abusing kids, or for those who are currently wards of the penal system. However, the vast majority of the kids we meet are somewhere between immediate, life-threatening danger and ordinary life, and in today's teen world, ordinary too often equals dangerous. We need a perspective and tools to handle this.

About the Examples

Hundreds of real-life examples are offered in these pages. Even with this variety, I've included only those situations that have repeated themselves, only those lessons learned many times over. To protect confidentiality, I maintain the same standard I've used in several previous books, which has by now become common among writers in the field: cases are completely disguised or written as composites. The litmus test I use is that the person(s) described should not be able to identify themselves. Everything recognizable has been altered, while keeping the essence of the situation intact. To do this I have edited these pages literally ten times over, to make sure that basic truths are in place, but the privacy of those involved is protected. If I have erred in any direction it is to tone down some of the examples, because the signature event of a teen scenario is often so publicly outrageous it might leave a child, family, or clinician recognizable.

Background

The relational–behavioral therapy approach suggested in these pages did not suddenly come into being for the purposes of this book. For 25 years I have been teaching and refining a model that integrates a powerful therapeutic connection in order to promote life-altering behavioral change. The synthesis evolved naturally as I became clearer about the new realities of 21st-century teens. The absence of sustaining adults in kids' lives at early ages, teens and adults living in often parallel worlds, the astonishing power of the adolescent culture, along with a weakening of the family's gravitational pull at home, made it clear to me that without a strong attachment to a guiding adult, kids will not take the risk to move toward healthier behavior and attitudes.

In the model I present, every aspect of a clinical relationship that I have found promotes an internalization of the therapist's voice or presence has been integrated: from the basic therapeutic conditions kids need to feel "held" in a modern therapy relationship, to the art of giving advice to adult-dismissive adolescents, to the use of counter-transference and self-disclosure that authentically provokes teens to take us seriously.

But relationship (and insight), are rarely enough. Behavioral change is essential in developing a strong sense of self. So, strategies that help promote effective behavioral change are also integrated in the model: from no-nonsense directives, to impassioned debate, to un-self-conscious inquiry, to dramatic role playing, to changing the parameters of the session, and much more.

It has also become clear to me that working with families or kids alone is meaningless, at best; at worst, it recreates the disconnected world of adults and teens today. Unfortunately, meeting with families is a daunting proposition to therapists who work with teens individually. At the same time, seeing kids alone is foreign territory for many family-trained clinicians. The truth is that family sessions with teens scare most child professionals, almost as much as they do kids and parents. So, included in these pages is a clearly articulated approach that I call "focused family sessions" —meetings that keep therapists in control, while challenging both sides of the generational divide—without threatening the empathic connections you've worked so hard to establish.

Impossible Therapeutic Dilemmas

Paradoxes we don't often talk about are built into treatment with adolescents. Certain dilemmas drive both parents and therapists crazy. They are given their due here, and include the following: handling the field's rigid rules about confidentiality that undermine teen treatment, lessening chronic lying to therapists by basically moral kids, staying effective in ordinary situations that hold us hostage and keep us at wits' end (especially during the springtime), maintaining the elusive balance between a teen's need to differentiate and a parent's need to know, what to do with "finding out" and then wishing you didn't have to deal with what you've learned, the disappointing sequence of presenting problems improving and then being followed by a worsening of the situation—as healthier kids find themselves more involved with high-risk but totally ordinary behaviors.

Such paradoxes are maddening to those of us who work with teens and parents. But this book is about trying to face treatment challenges squarely, coming up with practical and clinically sound ways of handling them.

A Warning and an Invitation

First, some of what I suggest is controversial. Do nothing that violates your sense of ethics, or state and agency regulations. Go over anything of concern with your supervisor—in the end it is your knowledge and judgment that counts, not mine.

Second, let me know what works and what doesn't. Teens are human beings in a process of growth and great upheaval all at once. Since the new adolescence is changing as fast as the world we live in, the feedback you offer helps refine this model, adding further coherence, as "kid-life" keeps morphing from year to year, even moment to moment.

Last, since I've worked with teens so long, I have been humbled many times over. I know that I don't know. I cannot tolerate the arrogance of clinicians who think they have all the answers. So it feels critical that we share what works and what fails. Let's face it: kids talk to each other all the time—online, through text-messages, using call-waiting, chilling, sharing the pop culture or TV—and adults do not. Compared to the intensity of teen communication, it is surprising how little the important adults in teens' lives speak to each other. We ought not be part of this collective grown-up ignorance.

Ask my publisher to contact me. Let me know what I've gotten right and what I've gotten wrong, and also what you've discovered along the way. In the end we need to be at least as informed as the adolescents we are supposed to be helping.

A final hope—this book was fun to write; it is not meant to be a heavy text, it is a mirror of experiences we have, or can have, with the new adolescence. These kids shimmer with life. In the end, they help us to be joyful, even as we help them through a new world of possibility and danger.

1

CONTEXT

The New Adolescence and a New Treatment Paradigm

Wazzup?

Johnny says I'm a faggot. I'll rip his arms out—then we'll see who's gay! Bitch! *How did Jenny get that tattoo? I'm going to throw up.* Just do it! *A lot of kids are going to crash that party.* Parents, the antidrug. *Mom will kill me— wait, I'm at Dad's this week.* Get the stuff! *I want Game Boy, I want PlayStation 2. . . .* You've got mail! *Wazzup! Hey, everybody does NOT think I'm bipolar!* New standardized tests. . . . *Shit, I don't get this math. The test's tomorrow, but first I have to check my e-mails and then listen to the CD I just burned and. . . .* Twelve more killed in. . . . *I'm so tired, but what's that noise outside?* Order in the next 30 minutes and. . . . *Mom, I am NOT too young for a thong!* New unemployment figures. . . . *Valerie's father died and Betsy's parents just split up and Bobby's family is moving away.* You're a teenager now, deal! *I just can't take it anymore!*

Get into the private thoughts and experience of enough kids today and it often sounds like they're coming apart at the seams. Teens and preteens pulsate in a pressure cooker youth culture and an explosive world, ever at the edge. Not that you'd notice this chaotic stream of consciousness when you first meet them.

Kids don't usually come in with raging guilt, repression, or conflict—the traditional, "gold-standard" symptoms of neurosis. They rarely present with posttraumatic stress disorder (PTSD) as their main complaint and, in fact, seem quite removed from the world-worries that media, parents, and trauma experts seem to focus on. Indeed, today's children and adolescents often present so convincingly they hide an entire world from adult eyes.

Lauren's mother, Margaret, loathed her 14-year-old daughter's weird new look—hair dyed bright orange, pierced eyebrow, Dracula makeup. But though Lauren looked bizarre and tended to stay out too late, she hadn't ever gotten into any real trouble. She was doing fine in school and seemed pleasant enough at home. Remembering the awful, screaming fights with her own parents as a teen during the '60s, Margaret tried hard not to antagonize Lauren and to be understanding.

Her determined empathy seemed to be working. When she asked Lauren in a carefully neutral tone why she wanted to look that way, her daughter good-naturedly tried to explain. Lauren described boys she thought were "hot" and even brought kids home to eat and watch TV. In turn, Margaret told Lauren about her own adolescence, and how she had yearned for freedom from rigidly moralistic parents, who were suspicious of her every move. Mom was still a little worried about Lauren's dramatic appearance and her late hours. But she was also proud of being the kind of with-it mother a girl could really talk to about what it was like to be young and busily exploring life. She thought that as long as the two of them could have such warm, open dialogue, nothing very bad could happen to Lauren. Margaret's dreamy vision of mutual trust exploded the day she came home to find her daughter in the bathtub having sex with two boys. Shrieking, she got the boys dressed and out of the house. Then, she confronted her daughter.

Lauren protested that the whole incident had been entirely innocent. "You must have been imagining we were having sex because *your* parents were so strict and you were wild as a kid," she said. "Besides, there were bubbles in the tub—how could you know what was really going on?"

For a brief moment, Margaret nearly fell for it—was it possible she had gotten it wrong? Then, furious anew, she asked, "What do you think I am—a damn fool?" "Yes," Lauren said flatly. Shocked and frightened, Margaret called the same day to arrange a therapy appointment for her daughter.

During the first few sessions, I learned several things about Lauren's life her mother did not know. She told me, for example, that she and her friends often smoked pot together, some of her buddies were heavy drinkers, and all engaged actively in sex— mostly oral or anal sex, which kept them, technically, "virgins." Not only did Lauren live much of her life in a world beyond her mother's view, she lied about it with virtuosity and shamelessness. When I asked Lauren why she couldn't talk to her mother about her life, she sighed and said Margaret became mysteriously un-hinged when she heard "about this stuff," particularly anything to do with her sex life. "My mom freaks out over anybody even think-ing about oral sex—I don't know why," Lauren said to me, in a genuinely puzzled tone of voice.

Lauren's story is not unusual. In my own practice and work-shops I present at around the country, I hear scores of similar stories about presumably "nice" kids and their responsible, hard-working parents—who seem to live in different solar systems. Ex-perienced counselors and teachers feel stunned and paralyzed, un-prepared by their training to deal with what looks like a completely new brand of adolescent. Like me, they have met children who have vandalized buildings without experiencing any guilt; talked with young teens who have sex in school bathrooms, not caring who walks in on them; and heard about adolescents who break into abandoned warehouses to hold "X-treme" wrestling matches that continue until one of the participants is left unconscious.

"I feel shell-shocked," says Alice, who has spent 20 years as a school counselor in Ohio. "Just about every Monday, kids come in showing off their tattoos. They tell me about gang bangs, binge drinking, raves, group sex in every possible permutation. And these aren't high school seniors, either. I'm talking about 13-, 14-, and 15-year-olds—and the most frightening part is that their par-ents haven't got a clue."

Researchers aren't terribly surprised, given upward trends in middle school and the first years of college, the lessening gap be-tween girl and boy high-risk activities, the increased use of mari-

juana, the debate on what kids now mean by the term "abstinence," as well as the normalization of binge drinking. This is not
to say that every teenager is hawking drugs, engaging in group sex,
or exploring new forms of violent behavior. In fact the latest
research on some benchmark high-risk behaviors—drinking, sexual intercourse, and teen pregnancy—seems to reveal downward
trends over the past decade ("2003 Youth High Risk Behavior Survey," Grunbaum, Kann, Kinchen, et al.). Nevertheless, you can vir-
tually guarantee that every teen who hasn't been home-schooled
since kindergarten or living in a house without electricity or e-mail
knows somebody who does engage in these behaviors. It is also
sure as taxes that a teen is not revealing a tenth of what he or she
sees or experiences.

So What's New about This?

One response might be, so, what else is new? Since when, during
the last 40 years, have American teenagers *not* evaded the gaze of
adults, incensed their elders, and inspired media melodrama about
juvenile outrages? Isn't "bad" behavior the birthright of adolescents?

I would like to turn this question upside down: *How could it be
that everything in our culture has changed so dramatically, yet somehow,
adolescence has not changed, that there's nothing new under the sun since
the time we grew up?* Does this seem even remotely possible?

The New Anxiety

*Spend time with teens and you gradually become aware that beneath the
jaded precocity and fearless acting out is a fretful undercurrent of worry
and fear, unimaginable for 11- or 15-year-olds just a decade ago. Get into
their daily lives and you will find thoughts racing, like overheated jet engines, from one source of stress to another—the next make-or-break standardized test, the next totally unsupervised after-school bash, the next late-
night, midweek concert they "have to be at." Explore a little further and*

you'll hear a palpable dread about going online with kids who regularly torment them. You'll feel their agitation about whether they should have sex after school. You'll catch the gnawing concern that their parents may break up, like so many others, or suddenly move the family halfway across the country.

* * *

Over the last decade or so, I've talked to thousands of parents, kids, and professionals across practically all regions and socioeconomic groups. To gain insight into this phenomenon, I began an informal research project. I interviewed more than 250 kids, pre-K through high school. I also met with kids and their friends in therapy and spoke to thousands of parents, counselors, and teachers. I spent hundreds of hours with young clients listening to their favorite music, reading e-mails together, and leafing through teen magazines, comic books, video game manuals, and student-run newspapers. From all these sources, I've gotten the same message: *Kids everywhere are overwhelmed by a tidal wave of culturally induced anxiety.* There's not a town or city—unless it's completely free of rapidly morphing family configurations; frenetic overscheduling; 24-hour, 500-channel TV access; and unlimited cell phone and Internet connections—that doesn't exhibit signs of epidemic anxiety among its youngsters.

What we used to refer to as the "presenting" problem, which presumably masked the real, underlying issue, has become something that requires less clinical detective work: *Often the real problem is handling the stress of normal, everyday teen life.* Fifteen-year-old John has been drinking too much and ends up in my office. Yes, his drinking is a troubling concern, but not compared to the viselike grip he feels about 30 hours of homework a week, four hours of basketball practice every afternoon, three hours a week of community service, and, of course, two parties a weekend. What about Julia, who's in therapy because of her almost-failing grades? Sure, she's worried about school. But what really preoccupies her is the phenomenon *The New York Times* recently called the "whore wars" (Guy Trebay, 2003). She's caught in a bind. She feels she must show as much skin as possible, but how can she do this when she's obsessed by the fact that so many parts of her body are "absolutely grotesque?" Of course, girls have lived with impossible standards of physical perfection for decades, but now it's happening at younger and younger ages—Julia is 11. And her friend Ethan, also a preteen, is one of the growing numbers of young boys I know who are obsessed about their bodies, too—not buff enough, too skinny, too small. "Might as well be dead."

Thirteen-year-old Peter is in my office because he's isolated and he turns people off. What's really going on beneath his haughty presentation, though, is that he's been typed as gay. Why? He once put his arm around another boy in a moment of friendship, and, since then, he's been accused of being "ass hungry." Mona's got it all—the perfect look, the perfect body and she's supersmart. So, what keeps Mona so fearful? Precisely because of her magnetism, she's the object of anonymous Internet insults, online come-ons, and, lately, direct threats on her life. What keeps Michael up at night is that he can't turn himself off after an ordinary evening. What's ordinary? Being online with six people at once while talking on the phone with two friends via call waiting, burning a CD for a pal, doing his homework with a friend, and listening to the TV in the background—just "to keep him company."

Don't reflexively blame their mothers or fathers. Most of these kids have reasonably responsive, competent parents, who feel as helpless as their kids about how to lessen the grip of this half-crazed pressure. After all, they live their own version of the same bind, stretched to the breaking point by their impossible work schedules and gut-wrenching economic worries. Parents feel hard-pressed to soothe themselves, much less their kids, from external pressures that have essentially colonized the family.

The New Anger

"Express yourself!" "Think it, write it, send it. Now!" "At least my parents aren't involved in a vicious divorce the way yours are!" "You think you're special just because you mother died?" "Don't come to school tomorrow, if

you plan to stay alive." "You're fat, you're bulimic, you're a loser." Mean Girls . . . Bad Boys . . . "Hey, is that any way to talk to your therapist?"

* * *

From playground back talk to schoolyard mean talk to high school rap talk to online death talk, casual communication between kids pulsates with a verbal brutality that makes adults wince. And this carries over into the home, where many parents tolerate enormous abuse from kids because they're frozen in place by 30-year-old pop psychology bugaboos: If kids aren't allowed to freely express themselves, they won't develop proper self-esteem. Kids today are verbally abusive, not so much from deep, festering rage or rebellion, which might once have been the case, but because they genuinely seem oblivious to the impact of their own actions on others. They've never been taught that what they do and say actually matters, that laser-like one-liners can deeply wound people. And when you don't have to face the person whom you insult—cell phone, beeper, e-mail—it's even easier to do. As one 12-year-old told me, "I can say anything I want online because I don't have to see how it makes the other kid feel."

The casual expression of anger starts young. Jessica has just been told by her mother to stop watching TV and clean up the table. "Not now," Jessica says, without bothering to look up. "No, Jessica, I mean this minute," her mother says sharply. "Later," Jessica responds, almost absentmindedly. Mom stiffens and threatens: "Stop it now or there won't be TV tonight." Finally, she's got her daughter's attention. Jessica looks her mother squarely in the face and says, "Fuck you, Mommy." Jessica is eight years old.

Fuck you, Mommy! The exhilarating horror of this phrase. How many adults today can imagine the consequence had they thought, let alone said, such a thing when they were kids? Over the last 10 years, however, as these exchanges are increasingly part of everyday family interaction, it has become apparent to me that a basic shift about acceptable behavior is taking place in parent–child relationships throughout the country. After all, Jessica is not a neglected or abused child in thrall to gang culture. Her parents live in a comfortable suburb. Nor is Jessica "maladjusted" psychologically; she knows her parents love her, she earns good grades in school and basically gets along well with other children. What's really shocking is that exchanges like this are so ordinary, they are a part of daily family discourse in America, even before adolescence.

A father informs me that his eight-year-old son, when asked for the fourth time to turn off the computer game and straighten his room, snarls," Leave me alone, butthead!" A 10-year-old girl, told by her mother to finish her homework, barely glances up, utters under her breath "What an asshole," and continues to play. I hear the "flailing tantrum" story over and over; a parent directs a child not to chew gum or to stop playing and get ready for bed; the child responds by hurling him-or herself at the parent, flailing away with small fists in a frenzy of anger. One therapist told me that a girl he had been seeing expressed her jealousy of an unborn sibling not by the usual array of anticipatory anxieties, but by smashing a baseball bat into her mother's pregnancy-swollen belly.

It is not just parents who are feeling the brunt of the explosive defiance that seems to be spreading through the ranks of American children. I remember attending a softball game led by an experienced coach, and watched it turn into a free-for-all. One seven-year-old, enraged after he struck out, grabbed home plate and ran off in a howling tantrum; another child, tagged "out," physically attacked the boy who had tagged him; a kindergartner, when she was called out by the umpire, ran up to him, screamed "I hate you," and actually kicked him hard three times in the shin. All this in a friendly neighborhood game for kids and their families.

In interviews with important, nonparental adults in kids' lives—teachers, coaches, principals, community leaders, camp owners—I've heard about the same disturbing pattern of anger and even disdain for adults. One eminent children's theater director says that in 25 years of producing plays, he has seen increasing disrespect for him and his colleagues by his young charges. "I can't describe the enormity of change in the way children behave. I can no longer count on having their respect and attention merely because I am the adult and a teacher—now half the struggle is just to get them to listen to my directions." Even therapists are taken aback by breathtakingly raw affronts to adult authority. Expert clinicians have told me that it is not at all unusual for grade or middle school students to look them dead in the eye, say, "Who do you think *you* are?" and then get up and march out of the session.

The New Parenting Confusion

What do fathers and mothers do these days when their young child curses at them or goes into a flailing tantrum or daily beats up a younger sibling? Not very much, as it turns out. Speaking for many, Melanie described her reaction when her six-year-old son, Eric, hit her and screamed at her in the supermarket: "I didn't know whether it was better to smack him on the spot or let him get his feelings off of his chest so they wouldn't fester." Other parents respond with intense rage and unenforceable punishments. In the face of her daughter's "Fuck you," Jessica's mom immediately spanked her and threatened, unconvincingly, to take all TV away for a whole year. Several weeks later, while watching television together, another version of the same incident occurred.

* * *

Parents have become so anxious about doing the *wrong* thing that they often become paralyzed. For example, 10-year-old Mindy had been invited to a party one night, where, she said, the kids would be playing make-out games. "What should I do," Mindy asked her mother, Ann, "when they start kissing?" But Ann was as unsure as her little girl. Finally, after what seemed like endless hesitation, she offered, "In the end, it's whatever makes *you* feel comfortable with who you are," a wishy-washy, unsatisfying answer that left Ann discouraged and Mindy very annoyed. Later, Ann confided to me that she didn't know what would be better, letting the child "harmlessly" explore her emerging sexuality or setting strict limits that she might rebel against—and choose not to confide in her next time.

Bill, the father of depressed, 13-year-old Jason, was in an equally serious quandary. After a couple of lonely years without friends, Jason had finally found a buddy—a classmate he brought home during lunch period. The tentative friendship seemed a real breakthrough, except for one tiny detail: The two boys spent the lunch hour in Jason's room smoking dope. Should Bill ignore the infraction of school policy, not to mention state and federal drug laws, in relief that his son found a new chum? Or should he crack down on this illegal and dangerous behavior? Which was worse for the boy—being a friendless and possibly scapegoated loner in school or a budding pothead with a pal?

Adults are not only confused, they often seem to have lost their own moral direction. What, for example, happened to Chrissie, who screamed at the umpire and kicked him in the shins at the Little League game? Incredibly, her mother, who was watching, did not reprimand her. The umpire did not kick her out of the game, and a few minutes later, Chrissie got the weekly achievement certificate she'd "earned"—a red ribbon for her participation.

Moral relativism also seems to have become the collective attitude of what I call the "second family"—the kid world of peers and pop culture—that is often more important, and more visible, to children than the " first family" of their parents and siblings. Although the younger children I have interviewed—five to seven years old—strongly believe in right and wrong and are angry when their parents fail to set rules, by fourth or fifth grade they begin talking in ominously relativistic terms about moral issues. Much to the dismay of adults, many children, responding to events like schoolyard murders, make remarks like "I don't think what they did was right, but I don't completely blame them either. They were treated badly, and anybody can crack under certain conditions."

In 1996, the *Rockford Register Star*, an Illinois newspaper, gave us a glimpse into the second family's code. The newspaper polled hundreds of teens in heartland America, asking them what moral guidelines they followed. "There aren't any," these kids answered almost unanimously. "You only need to treat others the same way they treat you." Almost none of the teenagers, boys or girls, were prepared to label any behavior, no matter how noxious, simply right or wrong.

More disquieting, and perhaps more instructive, few of these kids had ever considered that adults might in some way be able to guide them in making decisions about issues of right or wrong.

And why should they? Most of the grown-ups in their lives don't understand the details of second-family living or believe in their own ability to redirect their children—a failure kids pick up on only too well.

The Maze of Modern Childrearing

In truth, the cyclical waves of often contradictory advice thrown at parents over the past 30 years may be part of the confusion. As parents scramble to do what works, they try out the latest one-size-fits-all theory, only to find it superseded by a new popular orthodoxy. Parents get hooked on different childrearing techniques, which tend to swing crazily back and forth between poles of permissiveness and toughness, regardless of whether these off-the-rack approaches are actually appropriate for their individual child.

*   *   *

Alessandro, for example, had gotten into another bruising battle with his little brother, who screamed in pain. His mother, Hillary, tried an approach based on Thomas Gordon's parent effectiveness training (PET) Using "active listening" techniques, Hillary asked open-ended questions to help her sullen boy express and neutralize his feelings of jealousy. The more she employed this kind of therapy-speak, the more tight-lipped he became. "Oh, forget it," Alessandro finally said in disgust and walked away.

The "tough love" approach, with its emphasis on setting limits and quashing what was felt to be too *much* expressiveness, is where 12-year-old Jenny's parents decided to put their money. Jenny had been drinking and hooking up with lots of boys, staying out way past her curfew, and doing poorly in school. Her father, Bob, already overly rigid, treated Jenny to an ironclad lecture on bottom-line consequences. Days after his fire-and-brimstone sermon, Jenny didn't come home at all, having found a place to crash with some loosely supervised kids in the neighborhood.

As knowledge of widespread family abuse and incest surfaced during the late '70s and early '80s, the pendulum in childrearing advice swung back toward empowering children. The "self-esteem movement" was born, encouraging both parents and children to believe that every child was special for just being a person.

Part political, part reaction to inexorable increases in childhood disorders and acting out, the self-esteem surge was soon overtaken by an even bigger wave, emphasizing "family values." During this period, parents were advised that if they taught their kids morality, psychology would take care of itself.

During the early and mid-'90s, neurobiological discoveries caused the tides to shift once more in favor of the biological underpinnings of various childhood difficulties. And, most recently, in reaction to this biological trend, regarded in some circles as a flimsy mechanism for providing alibis to undisciplined kids, authoritarianism is making a comeback. "Children should be punished for every act of disobedience, no matter how small," intones John Rosemond, a main spokesman for the new movement. Spanking is highly recommended by the tremendously popular conservative psychologist, James Dobson. Is it any wonder parents and professionals are confused?

The New Anonymity

"Sometimes," says one of the preteens in my study, "I get the feeling my parents don't know me." "Mine, too," yells an irate classmate from across the room. "We don't spend time together—we're always so busy in my house." Just about every child nods enthusiastically.

*   *   *

It is logical that many parents buy great quantities of off-the-rack advice, because, stretched to the limits as we are, we do not always know the children we have. We cannot always tell the ways in which our kids are uniquely different because we just do not spend enough direct, one-on-one time with them. The hard truth is that most parents deeply love their children, but they don't protect enough time to pay attention to them. They do not really hear them. They do not really see them.

This sounds harsh, and it is a bitter pill for overworked mothers and fathers to swallow, particularly those who feel their lives are already intensely child-centered. Indeed, there is research from the Kaiser Family Foundation indicating that parents today spend the same, if not more, time with their families than June and Ward Cleaver ever did. But when Kaiser examined the kind of time families spend with one another ("Kids and Media at the New Millennium," Kaiser Family Foundation, 1999), we get a troubling picture of what so-called family togetherness actually looks like these days. Family members may be spending time *near* each other, in the same house, but are engaged in parallel yet separate activities, and not even remotely doing things together. Indeed, a long-distance phone conversation can provide a much closer and more intimate experience of connection than a typical evening in the bosom of a modern American family. Mother, for example, may be supervising her five-year-old in the bath while calling work to arrange a meeting for the next day; Sister is e-mailing several buddies and talking with yet another friend on the phone; Dad (if he lives at home, or if it's his weekend with the kids) is busy doing a report or watching TV, looking up every 10 minutes or so to announce "It's nearly bedtime" to whatever child might actually be listening.

What happens to children when they do not get the kind of direct, undivided, personal attention they need from their own parents? When they lack confidence in the capacity of their own parents to guide them? Where do they look to find something that promises to assuage their yearnings for attention? Nature abhors a vacuum, and for American children, the great, roaring hurricane of the mass media culture—particularly the culture of celebrity—rushes in to fill the psychic void that family used to fill.

The Culture of Celebrity

"What do I wish for? That I could visit Shaquille O'Neal or that he could come to my house." Twenty years ago, I rarely heard about celebrity fantasies in my work with kids; now, I rarely don't. Increasingly, children answer my questions about what they would like most by stating that their greatest wish is to be near a celebrity.

*   *   *

This is sad, but less ominous than the hunger within many kids to achieve celebrity status themselves, as if this were the one best bet for achieving the attention and sense of being known that seems to elude them. For too many of the kids I interviewed, the lesson of a tragic schoolyard shooting is the celebrity given the shooters. Highly visible events are ultimately successful, say many children, because dramatic acts make one instantly famous. Perhaps in a celebrity-drenched culture, most of us occasionally want to be famous, but for children who are furious because they cannot always get the personal attention of the people they love the most, the desire to be seen can become an all-encompassing and toxic need. In a medium of fragmented families whose members live parallel lives, in which children often feel more catered to than truly known, where off-the-rack childrearing techniques complicate more than they resolve and moral relativism is the norm, the culture of celebrity is a potentially inflammable ingredient.

Kids who commit public violence or wild acting out have found a metaphor that describes the pain of, as well as the solution, for their invisibility. They engage in such behavior precisely because it makes an unknown child uniquely recognizable. In a vulnerable child's mind, violence or outrageous behavior appears to be the perfect antidote to the anonymity of his or her life.

The New Wall of Silence

Even more striking than dramatic adolescent behavior is this: The silence kids always tried, with limited success, to maintain in the face of adult prying has become a reality—a great wall they have actually built between themselves and adults.

*   *   *

While kids have always lied to adults, never before have they lied with such ease, confidence, and lack of fear or remorse. Because of the distance between themselves and adults, they can afford to lie without qualms because they realize they are unlikely to get caught. Unsupervised by overworked and overstressed parents, living in communities where neighbors are strangers to one another, attending large, impersonal schools where teachers may not even know their names, they "get" that adults are hardly aware of their existence, let alone what they are doing. How could this be, when today's parents seem so committed to proactive child-rearing?

Today, the diminishing gravitational pull of the first family (the nuclear and extended family at home), for decades apparent in urban populations, has finally become palpable at all socioeconomic levels. Trends begun in the '70s have dissipated the power of the first family. As we all recognize by now, divorce (50% of marriages), mobility (about 15% of the population moves every year), and economic pressures that generally require both spouses to work ever-longer hours have undermined the old stability of the family. The "traditional" configuration of male breadwinner and wife at home fits only a tiny fraction of today's households. Time-squeezed parents even in intact, dual-earning families have few moments to spend with their children. Though his figures are open to debate, MIT economics professor Lester C. Thurow wrote in *USA Today* ("Changes in Capitalism Render One-Earner Families Obsolete," January 28, 1997) that parents now spend 40% less time with their children than they did 30 years ago, and two million children younger than 13 have no adult supervision either before or after school—a figure which has recently moved even higher.

Furthermore, the family's informal support systems—the extended kin networks, church and community organizations, PTAs, and neighborhood ties—that buttressed family life have gradually disintegrated. For example, PTA membership since 1964 has fallen. And while Main Street, with its network of well-known shopkeepers and familiar customers greeting one another every day is too often deserted and half boarded up, huge, impersonal malls on the fringes of town are the real center of urban and suburban life in the United States.

Into the void left by the withering of adult community life has rushed what I call "the second family," the vast wave of adolescent peer groups and pop culture "out there." Their influence has been hugely expanded and energized by a technological explosion that has proven its power to blast into every home. Two-year-old children, without developed language ability, can recite the McDonald's jingle; indeed, researchers have found that 18-month-old kids are already capable of brand-name recognition. Despite what your friends may admit, the average high school graduate has spent 15,000 hours of his or her life in front of the TV, compared with only 11,000 hours spent in school.

Perhaps nothing reflects the profound changes in teens today, or demonstrates distance between the generations, as much as the online invasion. Never before have so many kids spent so much time directly in touch through electronically mediated worlds uncontrolled by their parents. Online, as so many kids have told me, they can assume different identities, personalities, genders, ages, become anyone they like, and interact with hundreds of chameleons doing the same mental shape-shifting—and they can do it all without parents being any the wiser.

One mother said about her 14-year-old daughter, "She's online every day with friends whom I've never met and never will meet. Five years ago, I might have at least spoken to some of them on the phone when they called, but now, I don't know who they are, or what they talk about or where she goes with them. Unless I literally sit down with her every single time she goes online, I have no idea what a very large chunk of her life is like, or even who she is." This vast, unsupervised world of the Internet *is* something new under the sun, and it is not only transforming the way kids live their lives, but also the way parents experience kids—or fail to experience them.

The most significant relationships many of them have is with one another—and with the vast corporations that sell them $160 billion worth of music, clothes, electronics, and sporting goods every year. As Deborah Meier, education reformer and MacArthur Fellowship winner, writes, "Who besides the people who organize the marketplace for our young . . . is keeping company with our kids? Who else is observing them closely?"

Parents are further distanced because they have bought in to the implicit ideology of the youth culture: Kids are a world apart, with rights to complete freedom and independence from adults. There is a scene in Philip Roth's 1972 novel, *Portnoy's Complaint*, in which the beleaguered protagonist, talking to his analyst about his mother, says there wasn't a crevice in the whole house she didn't know about, including every crevice of his own body. How times have changed! Today, many adolescents assume a natural entitlement to privacy: The "adults, keep out!" signs of a former era have been replaced by a padlock on their doors to do whatever they want within the confines of their own sanctum. No wonder kids feel confident they can live and lie behind an almost seamless wall of silence.

The New Compassion

When I get to really know kids, though, I discover they still need what young people have always needed: nurture, appreciation, clarity in expectations, and a sense of belonging. The tragedy of our times is that most adolescents do not get these basic needs met by adults and do not feel truly "at home" within their own families. If we are alarmed by the state of adolescence today—and I believe we should be—it is not because kids are lost souls, but because the kids we see have drifted out to the second family to find what is missing in their lives.

* * *

Noticing a group of young, teenage girls walking with their arms entwined or baggy-pants boys skateboarding, most adults can understand that the second family provides nurturance to kids. Kids, despite the rawness of life within the second family, hold each other to surprisingly tough, even harsh, expectations and rules of behavior. Sophisticated topics around manners, morals, and ethics unexplored by teens in earlier times are discussed and debated strenuously: how to initiate and end romances, what friends owe one another, how to regard infidelity in love relationships, and when and whether to share confidences.

Once the code to their behavior is cracked, it becomes clear that they are not all what they seem to their horrified parents.

Once they begin to trust, they reveal themselves in yet another surprising way—*capable of compassionate behavior that we would have
found unthinkable during our own youth*. I have witnessed hundreds of
teens—considered amoral and contemptuous—be kind, loyal, gen-
erous, and, yes, even moral when they are with their peers. Despite
media hype, the teens I see exhibit a real capacity for compassion,
tolerance of one another's personal foibles, and common sense. Indeed, in some respects, they seem far more advanced in the art of
friendship than we were at their age.

Sixteen-year-old Brett, for example, whose mother called her a
"selfish, sarcastic bitch," had a reputation for being a wise guard-
ian angel to her friends. She encouraged one friend, whose father
was hitting her, to call an abuse hotline and sat encouragingly with
the girl while she made the call. She offered the guest room in her
house to a boy whose mother was often drunk when he came
home. On behalf of a friend who showed signs of bulimia, she organized several other girls to go to a school guidance counselor.
Without divulging the girl's identity, they asked what they might
do to help "someone who might have an eating disorder."

Brett is not unusual in her demonstration of openness and
good sense in her handling of complicated relationship issues. Because they have grown up in a culture suffused with the language
of therapy, kids talk to one another with more candor, intimacy,
and sophistication about everything—relationships, feelings, sex,
psychological problems, moral issues—than we ever dreamed of at
their age. Since 14-year-old Tony realized he was gay, he has been
enclosed in a cocoon of supportive friends. And, while he endlessly
discusses the complexities of gay and straight love relationships
with chat room buddies, he may also be helping another online
friend with her homework. In the meantime, he is known among
his peers as a good mediator, and regularly helps settle fights, such
as one between Marcia and her boyfriend, John, after she was
caught cheating on her exams. He also recently dressed down a
friend for spreading malicious rumors about a classmate, while
helping another prepare for an important audition.

Not only are kids more knowledgeable about relationships
than we were, they are much more inclined to break down tradi-

tional boundaries between males and females. In spite of the viciously sexist lyrics of some pop songs, close friendships between boys and girls in the second family are far more common than during our adolescence. Both sexes watch the same TV teen psychodramas—and learn the same language of relationship and feelings. While girls are still more emotionally expressive than boys, the gap has narrowed, and kids seem to draw "best friends" almost as much from the opposite gender as from their own.

Consider 13-year-old Tamika. After her parents divorced and her older sister got married, she became increasingly despondent, something she hid from her mother, along with her nightly habit of raiding the liquor cabinet. When Mom brought her in to see me, I asked her who she would most trust if she needed help. To my surprise, she answered, "Tommy and Kirk. They're my closest friends." In fact, it was Tommy and Kirk who broke the wall of silence between adults and teens in Tamika's life, alerting her mother about the seriousness of her situation. "Mrs. Washington," they said to her, "we're scared that Tamika might do something bad to herself."

If peers seem to be providing some sort of reasonable facsimile of family life, why not just let kids raise themselves? Recently, one mother admitted to me that she thought the peer group was practically raising her 16-year-old son. "If I'm honest, I'd have to say that with both his father and me so busy, we really don't have time to give him much guidance—so his friends are doing it. In some ways, I don't think they are doing such a bad job."

But our society has never formally thought children should be left to stumble along to adulthood unaided and unguided by their elders. However sophisticated teens seem, they don't magically become grown-ups at 13. Neuroscientists have now learned that it takes about 20 years for the brain's prefrontal cortex to achieve the physiological maturity that allows for full impulse control. Adolescence is still a time of intense emotions and fluctuating identity, of absolutes and debilitating insecurities. Kids not only need the anchor of reliable relationships with adults in their lives, they secretly yearn for the kind of knowledge that mature people have acquired through years of observation and experience. Unfortunately, this combination of relational need and need for adult guidance is exactly what they aren't getting from us.

A New Paradigm for the New Teen

Fifteen-year-old Mary says, "I went to the guidance counselor because there are these kids who keep saying horrible things about me and threatening me. I can't avoid them: They're on the school bus, they're in my class, they're online sending me gross messages. I wanted to know what I should do. So what does the guidance counselor say? She says, 'Tell me what you think you ought to do.' Do you believe that? Why the fuck does she think I asked her in the first place? Is this supposed to be helpful? What is it with you people, anyway?"

* * *

Mary's complaint is well founded. Kids may be driven by their own concerns, but they are not stupid. For all their swagger, they know they don't know everything about life or how to grow up. Most teens still hunger (if just faintly) for a powerful relationship with a grown-up that facilitates both a deepening within and direction without.

As child professionals, who frequently find ourselves mediating between distressed parents and teenagers, we are better positioned than Mary thinks to offer kids and their parents what they need in this world. But to do so, *I believe we must reinvent the way we work.*

Should this really surprise us? When good kids act "bad," not to rebel, but to be seen; when kids in middle school engage in behavior once reserved for college students; when well-meaning adults feel hopelessly overpowered at home; when teens look great on the surface but suffer with extraordinary stress levels and anger internally; when gender roles shift—with girls as group leaders, boys as nurturers, boys and girls as friends—when new treatment techniques change as routinely as childrearing fads, we must reexamine what we take for granted.

Relational–Behavioral Therapy

Given the distance many 21st-century teens and adults feel from each other, your job is, first and foremost, to make a *relational connection* with the adolescent across from you. This relationship is absolutely essential for you to be felt and heard above the cultural din of teen life. *No traditional approach or narrowly defined, state-of-the-art protocol can substitute for such a connection.* In attempting to do this you may be, transitionally, the only adult in an adolescent's world who can have as much impact as the second family of the peer group and pop culture.

But relationship is not enough—you must use this connection to create true behavioral change in teens: less casual lying, a willingness to take your advice, the courage to try new approaches with peers and high-risk decisions, the understanding to deal with parents and other responsible adults in more empathic, respectful ways. *Your voice and advice become an ongoing presence in a teen's psyche.* "You are on my shoulder," says the adolescent, "I hear you even when you're not with me."

At the same time, the relationship, based on *"flexible confidentiality"* with an adolescent's mother or father, is a bridge to help adults know their child better, to become realists about the *"gray zone"* and therefore more effective. *Your understanding of development and 21st-century teen life allows you to offer specific, behavioral input and state-of the-art childrearing strategies.* Your ability to see kids and parents together, in what I call *"focused family sessions,"* and to use the relational traction you've already established, helps shift destructive dances that may have existed for years.

* * *

A *relational–behavioral* approach is a self-reinforcing cycle: You create an evolving connection with a teen and his or her parent(s). From this *relationship* you help move kids and adults toward *behavioral* change; the cumulative success of these changes slowly leads to genuine motivation and a strengthening of your connection. This, in turn, *creates greater openness and willingness to examine the* high-risk decisions of ordinary life that challenge kids, especially as their presenting problems diminish. Slowly teens and parents find more resources within themselves and are *less dependent on you and the second family* for definition. *Passion and empathy heal the "divided self" of modern adolescence,* allowing for other constructive relationships, un-self-conscious interests, and love to develop. At some moment along the way, almost unnoticeably, *you turn into a person of the past*—a comforting memory and a touchstone of practical wisdom for a young adult to hold onto.

Relational–behavioral therapy with adolescents is a new paradigm, and it requires a significant change of mind-set. The good news is that, much like adolescents themselves, we child professionals secretly do some of what is described in these pages. To do the work, though, we need an organizing paradigm that makes social-contextual sense—one offering new clinical perspectives and techniques that match how 21st-century kids and their parents actually live.

*   *   *

Ten Treatment Myths

In order to take on a relational–behavioral approach, child professionals must reexamine many traditional assumptions and turn "old-think" ideas on their head:

- The ageist belief that you need to be young, charismatic, and hip to work with adolescents.

- The unrealistic view that anything short of a powerful relationship, one that directly challenges teens to change behavior, will even be registered above the din of the special-effects culture the new adolescent lives in.

- The outdated notion that your role is to help kids separate and individuate from parents, rather than create greater connection between the generations.

- The false hope that as symptoms diminish kids get better, when, in fact, they often become worse, facing even more dangerous issues in the high-risk, "normal" world of the second family.

- The destructive commitment to maintaining an impermeable wall around treatment, rather than learning how to open up the relationship to parents, friends, and the deeply significant superficialities of pop culture.

- The myth that unconditional positive regard for teens can cut through their everyday lying and disconnection.

- The bureaucratic and theoretical belief that rigid rules about confidentiality protect, rather than undermine, the treatment relationship.

- The clinical bugaboo that concrete advice to both kids *and* parents will inhibit self-discovery or the development of genuine selfhood.

- The wrong-headed notion that specialization—working with children alone or just with the family—can heal the fragmentation in our culture.

- The omnipotent belief that seeing more than a few high-risk teens at a time is advisable—given the ongoing dangers of the new adolescence.

* * *

With everything up for grabs, the old model isn't enough. It doesn't work. And it's time to admit it. We need an approach that addresses 21st-century life, one that fits the new adolescents out there, as well as their beleaguered parents at home.

Even the first meeting requires something different than what we're used to.

2

FIRST MEETING

Getting Teens to Talk

With adolescents, sometimes the shortest distance between two points is a circle.

Decades ago, I did my internship at an urban teaching hospital. We spent a great deal of time learning how to do an initial interview. We were taught to start with the presenting problem and then go through a standard checklist of questions that helped us understand the "mental status" of the patient. One of the patients assigned to me was a very young man, Tom, who had been run over by a car during a psychotic episode. He woke up in the hospital gravely, although temporarily, injured. After Tom went through understandable rage at his bad luck, he was helped along in his six-month struggle by the sudden appearance of Deborah, a new patient on the ward. Tom and Deborah developed a relationship, and after a weekend pass spent together, they suddenly decided to marry. The entire ward was both thrilled and shocked that after this short time they would make such a big move. No amount of discussion with his fellow wardmates (who were quite vocal on the matter), the staff, and certainly me, the lowly intern, seemed to lead to any insight on either of their parts.

I called in my supervisor, Aryeh Anavi, and asked him to sit with us as Tom and Deborah discussed their future plans. For a few minutes I fumbled around, posing one lame question after another:

"How do you feel about your relationship?", "What do you think the reasons are you've been able to find each other now?", "How do your families feel?" and so on. Aryeh, with his usual impatience, broke in and took an entirely different tack, which went something like this:

"Tom, when Deborah's birthday comes around, what do you think her favorite present might be? Something that she'd really treasure." Tom was taken aback by this question about nitty-gritty "real life." He stumbled around a bit, and said, "Gee, honey, I don't really know. What would you like?" Deborah turned to him and said, "Anyone who knows me realizes that I love music." Not stopping, Aryeh then turned to Deborah and asked her, "Well, I heard Tom's been making a lot of headway in his recovery, and I wonder what some of the dinners are that you might plan for him. What is his favorite dish?" Deborah thought for a moment and responded, "Oh, lamb chops. I know that's what he loves." Tom looked and her and said lovingly, but with some disappointment, "No, it's really chicken."

There was a long pause. Aryeh then said, "So, what is it that the two of you really love to do together? What interests do you have in common?" Neither was able to correctly identify the other's particular interests. A quiet descended on the room until Tom said, "Maybe we're rushing into this too quickly. We know our problems, but maybe we need to know more about each other's everyday stuff before we get married. I guess this is what everyone has been trying to say."

Everyday Matters

I never forgot Tom's comment or the ease with which Aryeh had gotten this young adult and his girlfriend to open up, without ever asking a single question that seemed to focus on the traditional problem-centered inquiry. I was also struck by the fact that here was a young man who was known for being a very private person, one who had previously been impenetrable by even the best clinicians on the ward. These early lessons in one's training—part awe, part shame—often hold for a long time. Years later, as I struggled with the clients I met in our bustling emergency clinic in the heart of Brooklyn, I often thought of Aryeh's modest and highly effective method of getting young people to be straightforward. *Ask kids to talk about things that really matter to them.*

*   *   *

Many hundreds of clients and several decades later it became clear to me that some of the reluctance to talk on the part of adolescents had to do with my traditional approach. Times had changed; the kids I was now seeing did not have such specific problems. They were kids who had many behavioral or life issues more often than a single specific neurotic or borderline diagnosis. But, just as important, teens had become therapy-savvy. Whereas in the past I often faced clumsily mute, noncompliant clients, now, much more than not, kids were seemingly cooperative, glib, and even friendly to me. Yet as the interviews wore on, I realized that I was finding out absolutely nothing "personal" about their lives.

Matt, for example, was referred to me because he had been kicked out of several schools for not going to classes or doing his work and was on the verge of being suspended from yet another school. Matt's problems were typical of the changes I had noticed over the past two decades. He was a good-looking, bright young boy. He knew how to speak with sophistication about almost any topic and, on the surface at least, was willing to answer any questions put his way. The problem everyone—guidance counselors, psychologists, church leaders—had with Matt was that during an apparently successful give-and-take he revealed very little about his private thoughts, what his life was about, what could have motivated him to be so disengaged at school.

Somewhere around this time I made a basic shift. I realized that if we are going to understand adolescents, we need to adapt those first crucial interviews to how kids actually think today. Remember, today's teens are used to "climate-controlling" their emotional environment, to have things the way they want. The kiddie culture endlessly preaches that what counts is how they feel; the culture teaches them to be glib, but not necessarily expressive; the culture teaches them to regulate situations so they feel comfortable.

Taking all this into account, it became clear that Aryeh "got" a truth, especially applicable to adolescents today: We cannot be predictable, traditional, problem-oriented "shrinks." We cannot be the classic child professional most kids have seen so many times in the pop culture, have learned to take as a joke, and parry with so skillfully.

We need alternative ways to get kids to open up when we first meet them.

Interests, Not Problems

Regardless of a teen's or preteen's presenting problem, I immediately start our first meeting by inquiring about his or her interests in life.

I want to lower the level of a teenager's discomfort while paradoxically throwing him or her off the expectation that this will be yet another entirely predictable mental health experience. First, their discomfort: The quickest way to create painful silence or meaningless chatter in 21st-century kids is to push them onto a channel they can't change. Kids used to a remote control or a default key that allows them to surf through boredom or discomfort are not about to jump into uncomfortable discussions.

Interviews that rigidly focus on problems are precisely the wrong way to approach teens who are forced, remanded, or otherwise hauled into seeing an adult. By definition, most adolescents do not want to be with you, so they block the process with the kind of determination only teens can muster. Often, the number one question clinicians ask is *"Why were you sent here, what's your understanding, whose idea was it?"* To this question, you will hear versions of "they made me": the school demanded treatment, the court remanded it, my parents told me "I had to" and other reasons, boiling down to the notion that no *one in their right mind would do this willingly, rather than be with friends,* or be crazy enough to see a shrink. Essentially the door is already shut to openness. Thus, many kids, as well as those few kids who enter my lair voluntarily, need to grasp from the get-go that this experience will be different, not the one they've geared themselves up for.

If, as Freud believed, dreams are the royal road to the unconscious, in today's world, interests, passions, and pop culture pursuits are the royal road to a child's inner world. So I say, "OK, we'll get to the reasons you should or shouldn't be here later. *But, first, what are your interests?"*

Matt, whom I mentioned earlier, had been an abject failure in school and quite successful being expelled from one institution after another. It was not surprising that his main passion was video games. I asked, "What kind of video games? Tell me the names." Taken aback by this unexpected non-mental health question, Matt proceeded to describe an assortment of what I knew to be the most violent games on the market today. It was no accident that he could spend 10 hours at a time steeped in a world of killing, vengeance, and gore, because, as I got to know him over time, I saw that Matt's reservoir of rage was a primary reason he refused to cooperate with any of the schools he'd been sent to. The kind of video games he talked about in his first interview with me was an ordinary clue full of meaningful detail. Talking about this passion right off the bat signaled that our meetings were not going to be a predictable recounting of the same old tired story.

In another case, Lila told me that "eye-candy" movies were her only interest. These are the kinds of mindless teenage flicks that are "about absolutely nothing." Lila enjoyed sitcoms, hours of surfing TV, and "reality" shows. The depth of her shallowness was clear through her unbalanced interests. It came as no surprise that Lila's issue was maintaining relationships with peers and demanding pursuits. Lila was unable to connect with her own deeper feelings—enough so that even many of her school pals found Lila too boring to hang out with for more than a little while.

Pop culture includes movies, TV shows, and, certainly, music. Some time ago I purchased an inexpensive boom box to be one of my therapeutic tools. I invariably ask kids to bring in their CDs. I want to hear kids' favorite musicians and song lyrics. Obviously, one doesn't usually play music in a first interview, but it's important to find out what groups a teen likes, what performers matter the most, which lyrics speak to him or her.

In one such instance, it was very clear when I asked Ava, "What music do you listen to?" that she prided herself on alternative heavy-metal rock, so obscure it immediately set her apart from the rest of the girls in her suburban school. Ava had been sent to me because she was wildly idiosyncratic and could not fit in. She avidly nurtured this difference by choosing groups almost none of her peers could relate to.

Fourteen-year-old Kyle was depressed, chronically "dissed" in school, and developing serious psychosomatic problems. Why? Pretty simple, when you ask ordinary, pop culture questions. Kyle loved (the unthinkable for midadolescent boys)—show tunes! This taste in music, which he had shown during the elementary school years, inaccurately labeled him as gay, a mark he could not shake in the starkly homophobic teen world all around. Kyle loved show tunes, while his peers were into gangsta rap, trash talk, and jock posturing.

POP ED FOR CHILD PROFESSIONALS

As you listen to kids' pop culture tastes, it is essential that you actually have something to say. It may seem superficial or phony, but a 21st-century child professional is one who knows *a lot* about the pop culture world adolescents inhabit. As part of your preparation to effectively connect with kids, I urge you to check out the TV shows most adults reflexively steer clear of, believing (correctly) that they were not made for you. Take in movies you would naturally avoid, and become acquainted with music you may even have moral objections to.

As one precocious seventh grader told me years ago, "If you don't know what any of this is about, it's impossible to have an intelligent discussion with us." It is also far less likely that teens will open up to you, an alien representative from a distant cultural galaxy.

Licensing Exam Questions They Forgot to Include

1. Name five "reality" TV shows.
2. Describe the story line of one UPN, WB, or Fox melodrama.
3. Who "tells it like it is"? (a) Ben Stiller, (b) Hillary Duff, (c) Donald Trump, (d) Simon
4. What's the difference between gangsta rap and hip-hop?
5. What does POS mean?
6. Name the 10 teen movies that came out this past week.
7. Which TV star had her brother's baby?
8. Who is Usher?
9. What's on VH1 these days?
10. How many buddies can you IM at once?

Friends—More than a TV Show

After spending some time on pop culture tastes, I move a bit closer to emotionally charged issues. I ask who his or her friends are.

As I wrote in Chapter 1, there has been a profound change in the dynamics that impact on 21st-century teenagers. Over the past two decades, it has become starkly apparent that "the first family" at home often exerts far less gravitational pull on an adolescent (and sometimes on preteens) than "the second family" of the peer group and pop culture. As professionals who attempt to launch the process of change, we need to become aware of this second family. These friendships are often part of the reason a teenager has been sent to you in the first place; they also represent powerful resources for growth (see Chapter 10). Psychological conflict used to be considered the sole province of oppressive, dysfunctional families at home. Today, second-family dysfunction and second-family strength are of major concern, and they must inform our work.

Draw a "Friends" Sociogram

In order to help kids open up about relationships within the second family, I take a piece of paper and do a theme-specific sociogram. In this representation of the peer network, my client is drawn as a circle in the center of the page. I then ask, "Who is your closest friend? Tell me his or her first name. I don't want to know who he or she is, so just use the first name, please." I draw a circle placing that person closest to the client's circle, and then inquire about other friends. They are added on with varying degrees of distance from center stage. The sociogram we create together (in hundreds of cases, only one or two kids have refused) illustrates the basic terrain of the second family in a teen's everyday life.

Constructing this sociogram together lifts the curtain off an adolescent's world in a way that is easy and unforced. For example, as I wrote down Ava's different friends, we found ourselves crossing out one after another, or drawing one closer and then moving the same one further away. It quickly became apparent how second-family members continuously ebbed and flowed in their connection to Ava.

After doing this sociogram, it was equally clear that Peter had become deeply disconnected from school when his two best friends moved. For different reasons (one boy's father was reassigned to another part of the country, the other boy's parents divorced), each suddenly left. It was no accident Peter disappeared into the fantasy world of online video games; he could still stay in touch with these friends in cyberspace, while keeping his distance from the barren world of school.

Finding out the players in a teen's life is a good start. It is also important to inquire more deeply about these friends. An adolescent may be glib or sullenly reluctant to talk about him- or herself and yet be a pop psychologist or ethnographer when it comes to friends. I suggest asking these questions in a specific order having to do with their degree of intimacy—keep in mind the personal nature of peer connections. One enters any family with initial deference to privacy. It is no different with the second family.

Second-Family Matters

1. "What do your friends like to do?"

2. "Who shares your taste?"

3. "Where do you guys like to go out together?"

4. "Who likes to hang out with whom?"

5. "Who do you talk to online?"

6. "Who do you call when there's a problem?"

7. "Who's the best listener?"

8. "Who gives the best advice?"

9. "Who are you most worried about?"

10. "No names, but what are the substances of choice in your group?"

Approached in this gradual way, areas open up via talk about others. For example, it became clear that Drew had acquaintances. But he had no specific second-family person to talk to when difficulties came up. It was not a surprise that Drew was sent to me for his depressed, withdrawn state when, in fact, his peer group connections were so undeveloped. It was apparent to most other kids that Drew's friendship circle was sparse; but it was not so clear how much he missed a pal with a good ear. "Real boys" don't need real support, right? More about that later.

Julian, a much more peer-involved 15-year-old, was up every night with different kids in his second family, helping them through their endlessly intense situations. Julian's problem, unlike Drew's, was finding it difficult to remove himself from dramatic interactions—the rivalries, jealousies, and conflicts—that his friends discussed over the phone and online till all hours of the morning.

It is also possible to get into areas in the first session that are off-limits using the standard initial interview approach. I say this because in almost every first interview, I will ask the following;

"No names please, but what are the substances of choice in your

group?" The ethos of kids in different second families varies greatly, and other kids' choices are an indirect way for your client to discuss his or her choices. Mariah, a brilliant 16-year-old girl, had been coming and going without any curfew. This question led to an extensive discussion about the use of Ecstasy in her second family. Mariah let me know about her experience with "rolling"—a term to describe Ecstasy—by detailing how many times her friends engaged in this activity during the course of a week (pretty shocking, actually) and how extended use had gotten kids into serious problems that were still under the radar of adults.

Likewise, Stanley, a boy who eventually was discovered to have had a serious pot smoking habit, "told" me about it in the first session by describing the smoking rituals of his friends. Having broached the subject this way, Stan gradually let me know about his own daily smoking rituals.

Another of my clients, Charlene, a 16-year-old junior, revealed in our initial interview that she was adamantly against smoking pot, but made it clear that her friends were into binge drinking, and had been since the first year of high school. It was no surprise, of course, when Charlene quickly added that she, too, was a heavy drinker, but, "only on the weekends." This explained her weekend explosions at home, her slow crawl up from Sunday exhaustion to pre-Friday excitement, and her difficulty focusing for any length of time on schoolwork.

Leave No Teen Behind: School and Learning

By now, after "meeting" the second family, it is possible to bring up touchier issues—school and learning. Many kids who come in for treatment have undiagnosed learning or attentional difficulties. Since this is such a complex area, and may require psychoeducational evaluation, I use the first interview as an initial screening. Teens respond well to direct questions centering on ordinary school experience. Choose from these ordinary-life questions, which help sensitize you to undiagnosed learning issues, attention regulation disorders, and nonverbal learning disabilities:

Learning Issues Quiz

1. What are your favorite subjects?

2. Do you work more when you like a teacher?

3. Do you ever read for pleasure?

4. Do you put things off?

5. Do you work best under a deadline?

6. What does your room look like?

7. Is it easier reading textbooks or the computer?

8. Do you like to sit in the front or the back of the classroom? Do you ask questions in class or fade out?

9. Do you make errors on tests, homework, or reading instructions?

10. Do you edit your writing? Or once done-you're done?

11. Do you say or do things in class without thinking?

12. Are you uncomfortable in sports or good at them?

13. Are kids mostly nice to you or leave you out?

The "First Family" at Home

Perhaps 30 minutes into the interview I finally get around to the traditional area of mental health professionals: the client's family relationships. So far, adolescents have shared with me their interests, passions, day-to-day lives in school, and the players and dramas in the second family. By now one can almost feel pent-up demand to talk about the dreaded subject of life at home. You shouldn't disappoint. Though many kids are philosophically against openness with a child professional, they feel cheated not to have been "shrunk." Questions about the first family at home and what "landed you here in my office" now almost seem comfortable. This order of inquiry mirrors the way an adolescent views his concerns: second family comes first, first family comes second.

In this part of the meeting, I ask the following question: "What *annoys* you most about your parents?" For most clients between the ages of 12 and 17, the word "annoy" is like sodium pentothal. It immediately leads to divulging areas of conflict around the house as well as themes that may become part of your ongoing work together.

To this general question one often hears the typical responses. "My parents are crazy." "We fight about curfew." "She never lets me stay out as late as my friends." "They're always on my back about homework." "He doesn't understand," and so on. But "annoying" is a very well-known commodity to most adolescents, more evocative than therapeutic clichés.

Sam said that what *annoyed* him the most was not the way his father grounded him, or that he could never be sure his dad wouldn't lash out. It was because of his dad's gruff tone that Sam felt he could never really open up to him. What annoyed Katy was how her mother spoke to her in a kind of social work, "technique-y," manner whenever Katy brought up serious, sometimes life-and-death, issues about friends. For Eddie, annoying meant the times that his mother came home after a hard day's work and was too tired to even notice how trashed he was. To Paula, it was when her dad looked at her with a hurt expression on his face, and whether that meant the beginning of another depressive cycle for him.

After discussions through so many unexpected and even fun topics, the word "annoy" is a door that springs open into the near afterthought of life at home.

Customer Service: "How Can I Help You?"

Treating kids as sophisticated consumers, and defining your relationship as a service is necessary to move matters forward. Since millennium adolescents are adept at identifying needs yet often inept at meeting them, it makes sense to end a first interview with the question, "How can I help you?" Whether they have been remanded, coerced, or self-referred, most kids actually have some idea about what is missing from their lives. There is no downside to emphasizing your role as a helper, as long as it is accompanied by some recognition of your limits. "I don't know whether it will be possible, but I'll do the best I can."

In her prescient 1972 book, *Therapy in the Ghetto: Political Impotence and Personal Integration*, Barbara Lerner discovered that most families migrated from clinic to clinic—until they found a person who actually asked, "What do you need?" and *then* offered a relationship addressing that need. Hans Strupp, in his groundbreaking work *Psychotherapy for Better or Worse*, found a similar dynamic. People look for a relationship that answers their needs, and end the relationship when it either does or doesn't deliver. The idea that professionals cannot offer one standard, narrowly defined approach makes sense. Witness the limitations of rigid treatment—from orthodox psychoanalysis to "invariant prescription" to unidimensional PTSD protocols.

At the time of Lerner's and Strupp's work, the notion that patients could actually understand their own needs was revolutionary, though not surprising. I had seen too many adults precipitously drop out of treatment when therapists tried to force a particular school of thought onto them. Three decades later, the situation with adolescents is similar. Precocious teens often know what they want, but may be more helpless than we realize at effecting positive change. In addition, 21st-century kids from all socioeconomic levels are veteran consumers. Therapy is to kids (just as it is to most everyone else) a product that must ultimately deliver the goods.

For example, Lee told me she wanted to stop getting so annoyed at the kids in school. She wanted a best friend with whom she could spend time and confidences. We had gone over her interests, passions, peer network, drawn a map of her second family, described the drugs of choice of her acquaintances, discussed whom she spoke to in times of difficulty, and reviewed school performance and the areas of stress in her first family at home. All this created richness, a poignancy, when Lee said, "If you can help me keep one friend that I can tell things to, maybe I'll come back."

Ava—who had audacious tastes in music and other pop culture

Therapists Serve

1. What do you want to change with your friends?

2. What would you like to see different at home?

3. What would you like to change about yourself?

4. Let's pretend for a minute that I actually have the power to help you with any of this. What would you like to be different?

5. If you were to make three wishes, what would they be?

---

pursuits, was contemptuous of the patronizing tone her parents used "in order to make me feel more like an average American kid." Ava's intense self-consciousness in school had a different meaning to me, given the richly detailed picture of her everyday life that emerged in our first meeting. When I asked Ava what she wanted me to help her with, she said, "Make my mom talk normal to me; I already feel different enough in school."

And when Julian said "Maybe you could help me not feel so responsible for my buddies all the time," his request told a truth not apparent from his icy demeanor. After all, here was a boy who had just described the details of rescue missions on the Internet and phone, who was sacrificing his grades and health in order to be available to kids in even greater trouble. By interview's end, I knew just how dramatic his second family was—self-cutters, suicide risks, binge drinkers. I got what Julian's *real life* was about—far more complicated and dangerous than could be seen by adults' eyes.

What about Confidentiality?

The first meeting is coming to its end. A lot has been shared—usually much more than an adolescent may have intended. The issue of confidentiality is a natural one to consider, otherwise a teen may leave with an unexpected sense of vulnerability, one that often signals a quick exit from the relationship. But the perspective on confidentiality must fit 21st-century teen realities.

The usual therapeutic position is one that almost every contemporary high-tech kid is familiar with. By the time they get to us, many clients have been to several agencies and counselors. It's no news when professionals say, *"Anything you tell me is between us. But if I feel there is an immediate danger to yourself or to anyone else, that information will have to be shared."* The problem with this hackneyed statement is not just its predictability. Or that kids play at the edges of being truthful. Or that they tell adults just enough to make it seem as if they've been personal, but not nearly enough to help us understand what is actually going on in their lives.

The 21st-century context that forces us to reconsider confidentiality is the following: Kids and adults live in different universes. Rather than experiencing adolescent rebellion against enmeshment, many families suffer from lack of traction. Since most teens live with a "wall of silence" around them, adding another wall, this time around the treatment relationship, mirrors a basic problem raising adolescents in today's world. A helping professional is in danger of creating yet another parallel universe in which adults and children have little chance to get to know each other better.

Because the second family is such a powerful force, I now view confidentiality from a different perspective. The statement I casually make at the beginning of the interview (which often goes unheard), and then again toward the end of our time (when it has more meaning), reflects this perspective: *"If there's anything you **don't** want me to tell your parents, let me know."* The foreground and background are switched from the message "Except for immediate danger, this space is 100% private," to "This relationship is going to help you get more of what you want *and* help your parents become more effective with you." I continue: *"Anything you want kept just with me we'll talk about. I'll never say anything to your parents unless we've gone over it first."*

How do kids react? Most seem at ease with this agreement, figuring they've left out truly dangerous material anyway. At this point they still feel like they can manipulate the truth pretty much to their liking. Others completely forget what I've said the second they leave the room. Others are a bit concerned, but are willing to give it a try, especially since this first meeting has been so unlike what they expected beforehand. **A few can't accept this parameter.** In those cases I will discuss my reasons fully, but if it's still unacceptable I'll refer the client to a therapist who views confidentiality in a more traditional manner. This is rare—it happens once or twice a year. Kids have so much confidence in their wall of silence, are so sure of their abilities to dissemble (more on that in Chapter 6), that most are not too concerned.

In fact, just to show my respect for kids' ability to keep adults in the dark, I end most first meetings with the following question: *"On a scale of 1 to 10, how much of your life have you been honest about with me?"* The wry smiles and wide range of scores about their degree of honesty is a good way to begin an authentic relationship with an adolescent. Teens respect an adult who knows that he or she really doesn't know.

Recognizing our limitations is a great way to end first meetings. It is a welcome sign that this may, indeed, be a different kind of relationship than teens, living far off in their distant universe, are used to having with a grown-up.

3

FOUNDATION

What's Necessary to Build a Helping Relationship with Teens

> Without rules, there's chaos. I need easy times—pizza, watching a video, hanging out together. They don't listen enough to the stuff that matters to me! Get them to show their feelings—without bossing me.
>
> —*What 250 kids told me they need more of from parents and other adults*

Adolescents in the 21st century do not often have in-depth experiences with adults, yet the success of treatment rests squarely on the relationship you are able to create. Building this relationship with modern teens, however, must differ from narrowly conceptualized treatment paradigms.

First, working with adolescents in the ways I suggest is the most dramatic, edge-of-your-seat experience a therapist can have. In play therapy with younger children, for example, the therapist maintains a soothing tone and a comfortable, warm distance. The therapist observes and participates, often lulled into an almost trance-like state of fantasy engineered by the child. The purpose of this quiet acceptance is to help a child express his or her inner world as safely as possible.

In psychodynamic psychotherapy with adults, regardless of orientation, therapists maintain a variation of Freud's "evenly hovering attention," a process of letting one's experience float along with the patient's. Inquiry, reflection and interpretation are essential aspects of the work—which hopefully create an expansion of awareness, healthier ego functioning, and a relative balance in one's psychic life.

In self psychology, the therapist is "a mirroring self-object," which is a multifaceted effort to understand the patient as fully possible. Treatment creates an empathic relationship that was previously missing in the individual's life. The inevitable "repair" of a fragile empathic connection is based on a sense of respectful attunement and is central to the work of building more resilient self-esteem.

*   *   *

Unlike these inherently modulated approaches, the school of thinking that is most useful with 21st-century teens is the "relational" approach, derived from a synthesis of interpersonal and object relations schools. As I discuss later, a *highly modified* relational frame is particularly helpful with teens—the emphasis is on highly modified.

What the interpersonal–relational writer Darlene Ehrenberg calls *"the intimate edge of relatedness"* is a most helpful concept with adolescents (though Ehrenberg writes primarily about adults; *The Intimate Edge: Extending the Reach of Psychoanalytic Interaction,* 1992). By this term Ehrenberg means the ways the two participants in the room actually *feel* each other, the place where they touch each other consciously and unconsciously. The quality of this "edge of relatedness" is what differentiates relationships, because the edge varies so distinctly in feel and action from one person to the next.

Nowhere in clinical practice (except, perhaps, with certain affective disorders and borderline clients) is the edge as vital and demanding as it is with adolescents. Because of roller-coaster developmental changes, ordinary high-risk decisions, intense cultural pressures, and the chaos of teen living, adolescents demand a level of responsiveness that makes most of the approaches described earlier seem stodgy. They are, to use a favorite adolescent term, "old."

The relationship necessary is profoundly different from the

quiet acceptance of play therapy, from the evenly hovering attention of analysis, from the inquiry of interpersonal psychoanalysis,
and from the empathic mirroring of self psychology. It is certainly
different in its centrality from contemporary techniques, such as
PTSD protocols, eye movement desensitization and reprocessing,
coaching,and cognitive-behavioral therapy, to name just a few.

Your active participation in building a three-dimensional relationship is *essential* for teens to feel. They need to "get" that you are
right there, in the room, fully engaged and responsive. No wonder
therapists report that, when working with adolescents, you must
always be *on*. The edge of relatedness needs to be focused, flexible,
heartfelt, and multidimensional. Nothing less can create a relationship substantial enough to cross the teen–adult divide, to contain
the volatile nature of 21st-century teen life.

And, in order to build such a vital relationship, a number of
surprisingly basic conditions are necessary.

Rules

*"I'm sorry I'm late. Everyone was talking after school, I lost track of
time. . . . " "The bus broke down and I wasn't near a phone, so I couldn't
call. . . . " "We went to the pizza place and just hung out. . . . " "I thought
insurance was paying you directly. . . . " "There's a big reading test tomorrow, and I have to stay home and study. . . . " "You mean I have to pay even
though he had fever last night! . . . "*

*   *   *

These are just a few of the stories we hear from kids and parents about their therapy obligations. How do we respond? Not
well. For various reasons, most child professionals are progressive
and antiauthoritarian. In fact, when many of us began doing this
work, we believed our young clients' anxieties often resulted from
too many rules and too much rigid authority. Our training taught
us that a warm, fuzzy embrace was a godsend for children. At the
same time, many of us are again sensitized to constricting rules,
feeling overcontrolled by managed care, the Health Insurance Por-

tability and Accountability Act (HIPAA), and our own agency's bureaucracy.

Put it all together, and we are uncomfortable being rule enforcers. *But today's kids are in trouble partly because in their world there are so few rules that actually matter.* We need to recognize that despite our discomfort, a laissez-faire relationship is indistinguishable from the everyday chaos many of our young clients now experience.

Establishing clear rules creates the secure frame that teens and parents need to begin managing disorder in their lives. Addressing the concrete issues of commitment, setting priorities, and seriousness about the process brings to the surface issues that might otherwise undermine the relationship. Instead of skipping appointments or prematurely terminating, families held accountable start talking about financial concerns or other fears that are threatening to devastate the home. When professionals challenge a family's casual attitude about showing up on time, parents may begin to discuss the everyday chaos that can be so frightening to children. In addition, almost without fail, when a preteen or teen is late to therapy, the missed appointment time is used for the very problem that the adolescent has trouble with—substance use, after-school acting out, and so forth.

LATENESS, NO-SHOWS, CANCELLATIONS

When kids toy with the edges—lateness to sessions, missing a meeting—one traditionally thinks "It's grist for the mill"—what teens are expected to do anyway. Exactly the opposite is true. I've discovered, to my surprise, that kids are pretty much on time, often more so than adults. For the most part, they like to come to sessions. When that is *not* the case, our failure to address the issue almost always comes back to haunt us in serious ways.

If an adolescent who is usually on time is late for a session, I ask about it, reminding him or her of the rules: *"How come you're late? It's not part of our bargain. . . . So, what was going on?"* Rather than letting kids off the hook, I've learned to regard lateness as is a signal that something is being held back. Invariably, I discover that these few missed minutes of our session were the exact moments he or she was smoking up with friends, doing a quick drug deal, vandalizing property, or having sex for the first time. More often than we realize, kids arrive a little late and a little high—but not so much so that they can't carry off the meeting brilliantly. Again, this is the tip of the iceberg, a sign worth noting and discussing. Playing with the edges of treatment is often a way to tell us something extremely important is going on just out of sight.

When kids *miss* sessions, it is critical to address the issue—not just because of what it might mean in terms of resistance or an unconscious process. Sophisticated teens even use unconscious process in their own defense: "Didn't you learn in school that people forget stuff sometimes? Everybody forgets, it's just a Freudian slip. Go ahead—ask questions about my deep, dark unconscious!" Despite such bravado, chances are something *was* going on that caused him or her to skip a session. And, that something is often the exact reason the client is with you in the first place.

One boy, Marv, came in on a Friday afternoon saying he had to cut the session short and leave early to meet his parents for a family get-together. Instead of holding him to our time, I was the understanding therapist and said, "Okay, we'll end a little early." Next week I learned from Marv that he had arranged to meet several of his friends in the afternoon to go out and drink. They wanted to get a buzz on in preparation for a concert that evening, where they planned to get totally trashed. The short session was a telling indication of his extracurricular life—if I had paid attention. Friday afternoon? Meeting parents, not his friends? And what about that huge concert in the park just about everyone in town had heard about?

Treatment parameters need to be discussed and processed. During moments of dialogue around specifics, kids start to open up about what's really going on:

THERAPIST: Hey . . . it's not like you . . . you're late!

BILLY: Well, I was hanging with my friends, I lost track of time.

THERAPIST: You're usually very good with time.

BILLY: Well, stuff was going on. We were chilling.

THERAPIST: Who were you hanging with?

BILLY: Charlie, Ian.

THERAPIST: Oh, yeah, Charlie and Ian. They have later curfews than you.

BILLY: I know. It's annoying, they do so much more than me.

(In passing, Billy mentions that he and his pals smoked up just a little. This interaction about rules allows an opening behind the wall of silence.)

THERAPIST: OK, chilling and smoking up right after school. So, what's it like when you smoke?

BILLY: Cool . . . well, not always great.

THERAPIST: What happens?

BILLY: I don't know, it's kind of hard to put into words.

THERAPIST: I know. Kids have different experiences that they don't always talk about. Some kids get really relaxed, and some get a little self-conscious. Others get paranoid. Some kids don't feel anything. Do any of these fit?

BILLY: Yeah . . . I never thought about it, but I do get self-conscious, my heart starts racing. . . . It's even kind of hard to talk.

Ten minutes addressing lateness leads to a discussion that opens doors behind the façade.

Fourteen-year-old Craig was a seemingly nice boy who couldn't make friends. Like so many high-tech kids, Craig practically shimmered with underlying anxiety, which he tried to overcome by forcing himself into people's conversations—not a popular habit with his schoolmates. Craig and his parents were prone to cancel appointments at the last minute. After about the third time this happened, I reviewed the rules: They had to show up on time, and reschedule within 48 hours or be charged for the session. Reluctantly, his (very aggravated) parents began to talk about their everyday concerns. Mom had been laid off and Dad wasn't making enough to meet their expenses. In fact, meetings were cancelled at times when they didn't have the cash to pay for sessions. They felt humiliated and crushed by the pressure, and the situation wasn't at all helped by their son's increasingly expensive taste for the latest fashions.

We began by cutting Craig's therapy back to every other week, and then talked about what Mom might do to activate her job search and how they could reduce some of Craig's pop culture expenses. Enforcing these rules allowed me to continue building a relationship with Craig that might have been discontinued, like so many other adult connections in his life.

*   *   *

Concrete rules and your willingness to stand by them run counter to incessant contemporary messages about instant gratification. Rules protect the frame and provide reassurance that the relationship will not simply melt into thin air.

Rituals

A basic part of relationship infrastructure, especially for 21st-century kids, is the creation of dependable rituals that anchor adult–child discussions. Millennium teens *love* rituals, in part because they live in either an overscheduled vise or virtual chaos. It *is* surprising how much that sophisticated kid sitting across from you needs rituals so badly. Rituals had their place in how early analysts conceived of treatment. They helped create a safe container, soothing enough to counter the pathological force of the family at home. The idea, especially with teens, was to help a pry a child away from the neurotic maw of his mother or father. Routines were part of creating an alternate emotional space. This aspect of Old World psychotherapy is a valuable carryover into the 21st century. But the rationale for postmodern rituals is different.

♦ *Today's kids do not need to be pried away from oppressive family routines. As my interviews with children of all ages revealed, far too few rituals go on in their day-to-day lives.* Just about every child, regardless of age, brought up the lack of simple routines, "pizza and a video, hanging out, watching TV together." Modern life is so frenetic, parent and child are headed in different directions during the day and well into the evening. Even when today's family is home, family members rarely inhabit the same space—one is in the kitchen, one is online, one is surfing for a TV show to watch—and a teenager may be doing all of these at the same time.

♦ *The second family creates rituals that are missing in the homes of many kids.* If anything, the competing force we face is the second family, not home life. Creating a place in which a child shares personally meaningful rituals *with an adult* may be a unique experience for teens. Rituals strengthen the unusual: *a grown-up anchor and an alternative force to the grip of peers and tractionless homes.* Rituals also provide comfort for kids, a welcome pause in their daily schedules. Familiar treatment routines create comfortable predictability in a teen's life. And "comfort time" is exactly what the second family offers. This is in stark juxtaposition to everyday family life that often seems to be running off the tracks.

Old Can Be New Again

Twenty-first-century reasons for establishing old-fashioned rituals in treatment:

1. Makes kids feel less in the spotlight, less self-conscious.
2. Helps teens multitask-talk while doing something else.
3. Offers a path to their hidden concerns.
4. Allows kids to leave personalized "marks" on the relationship.
5. Provides the remnants of play for "grown-up-too-soon" teens.
6. Allows nonverbal communication for kids with language processing issues.

♦ *The content of rituals offers clues about what is going on in kids'* *lives.* Kids create specific rituals that matter to them. Rituals are not only a way of collaborating, but a way to express oneself. Significantly, a teen can express him- or herself not only through language, but nonverbally, which for many adolescents is much less demanding. Through rituals we learn about issues that are not easy to discuss, about secrets and second-family life that may be hidden by casual or careful lying.

Rituals are as varied as is the imagination. The best way I can illustrate the idiosyncratic genius of kids is through examples. Following are some routines that kids came up with themselves or that we created together. In preparing this chapter, I saw, again, how routines express security needs for a frazzled generation, while revealing issues that are hard to bring up in words.

HELLO RITUALS

Listen to the Lyrics

Elana, 14, made regular use of the boom box I keep in my office. Every week at the beginning of our meeting, Elana played new music for me. Her CDs opened up the week's meeting with a jolt—a world of alternative groups and bands. Many of the lyrics were incredibly offensive, graphically sexual, or aggressive. At first I didn't consider the music Elana blared on my boom box as conveying anything personal. But as I began to listen carefully, the lyrics expressed volumes about Elana's experiences of sexual harassment. A song from the musical *Rent* said it best—she'd become an object so compelling, every stroll down the street or the corridors of school challenged her boundaries and self-worth. The lyrics of many songs also alluded to problems secretly going on in her second family—histories of incest, self-cutting, depression. These words introduced me to details that troubled her every day. Music became an anchor for us, *and* a way to indirectly communicate content, without breaking friends' confidences or being embarrassed.

As I got better at understanding what the lyrics meant, Elana got better at trusting an adult with the pain behind her façade.

Security Check

Jonah, 15, arrived every week and began the meeting with a visual scan of the consulting room. Anything different would trigger his commentary—a book in another place, a new piece of mail on the top of my in-box, a pillow on the other side of the couch. This was Jonah's way to settle in, to make sure I was the same person he'd left the week before. Through this weekly security check, I experienced Jonah's vigilance–how much adolescent swagger masked his fear that people were not who they seemed to be. Jonah's powers of observation were well known by his peers and useful in his gambling and dope dealing endeavors. Vigilance was also about trust, which turned out to be the central theme of Jonah's family. Both his parents had long-term secrets that emerged during treatment.

"Dude, Check Me Out"

Sixteen-year-old Elliott was quite avant-garde. He wanted to make his mark as a hipster, a 21st-century Dylanesque figure, dressed in uniquely alternative outfits. So, each week, the first few minutes of our meeting involved me commenting on whatever combinations he had assembled—a tie with a sweatshirt, a somber, Western black hat with Bermuda shorts, or a Hawaiian-style surfing T-shirt with fake "nerdy" glasses. It was important for me to talk about his outfit because it was important for Elliott to be seen as someone entirely unique. From a large family, he felt overpowered by dramatic brothers and sisters. His second family was equally intense—creative kids in the artistic program of an inner-city school. Elliot's opening ritual with me, discussion about what worked sartorially and what didn't, turned our meetings into a place where he knew he would be noticed in an easygoing way.

"It's Tuesday, Where Have I Been?"

Teens normally have such packed schedules, with so much day-to-day drama, it's difficult to recall the previous week. Angelina, 13, developed her own ritual to help with this problem. She started meetings by sitting next to me and reading my notes from our previous session. Angelina needed to see what I had written, to make sure I got it right *and* to jog her memory, not surprisingly, since she had been referred because of chronic difficulty with schoolwork and plummeting self-esteem. Reading my notes not only captured the previous session, she could be *my* teacher, correcting *me*: my spelling, my impossibly bad penmanship. This was an especially comforting ritual because everybody lectured Angelina—teachers, quick-tongued friends, and, of course, her parents.

MIDDLE RITUALS

"I'll Talk—But Don't Look at Me"

Martin, 12, was chronically harassed by peers. In our culture of perfection, kids see everything—in Martin's case, a tiny limp, literally unnoticeable to me or any adult in his life. Martin's awkwardness from being relentlessly taunted had developed into excruciating self-consciousness, and my initial conversations with him were maddeningly halting. This was one of the other reasons Martin had become a mark for other kids. The currency of teen cool is quick repartee and easy dissing. No room for self-consciousness allowed. So the therapeutic spotlight was too intense. His single mother was understandably not happy to pay (even the clinic's sliding-scale fee) for a child unwilling to open up.

Then, one day, it suddenly changed. In my office I have a "stuffed" hedgehog, which oddly enough happens to be shaped like a football. Like many other kids before him, Martin picked up the hedgehog and threw it over to me. I tossed it back to him, and a lively "catch" began. From that moment on, the hedgehog toss became a staple of our meetings. The entire tone of treatment changed. Martin began sharing the issues that were disturbing him: "They were making fun of me in class, in front of the teacher"; "When I sat down at the lunch table, they said I couldn't sit there." Meanwhile, the hedgehog flew back and forth between us, our talk punctuated by related observations—"good catch," "nice throw," "not a bad one," "should you get that or should I?"

Without the spotlight, Martin relaxed and opened up to the relationship. One day the hedgehog was nowhere to be found. Martin's ability to talk was nowhere to be found either, until we spotted our football-shaped friend. Weeks later, when Dad came in for a family session, he was stunned at how comfortable Martin was. The simple catch had become our anchor in the room.

"Are You Thinking of Me?"

Fifteen-year-old Molly and I had rituals around food. Every week I ordered in a snack. And every week, part of the routine included me offering her some of my food. As the middle child in a family of three boys, Molly felt she didn't receive enough nurturance at home. She had been acting out her needs for more attention by drifting out into a second family of high-risk friends. They spent weekends secretly out at raves and underage clubs, hooking up with strangers.

Rituals are metaphors, often expressing a hidden truth. Once Molly declined my offer of food by saying "No, I'm good." I replied, "Molly, you make it sound like you're in a bar with your friends, because that's what people say when somebody offers them another drink." This turned out to be the opening—discussing how much to binge every weekend with her hard-drinking group.

"You Can't Make Me!"

Frank, 12, was also a kid to whom I offered food, but he never accepted it. The one time I *didn't* offer some of my lunch, though, Frank said, "Aren't you going to ask me if I want any food?" I replied, incredulously, "You never seem to want it." Frank shot back, "Yeah, but don't you have anything to give me?" "Sure," I said, "how about some of these crackers?" Frank's response? "Nah, I don't want anything." We went through this exact routine—me of-

fering, and Frank saying "no" every single session. Perhaps because
of the comfortable smile on his face, I knew not to stop offering.

Again, the ritual had personal meaning. Frank's mother was
gone much of the time because of several jobs. To make up for her
frequent absences, Mom offered him things. Frank always accepted
these presents, even though they never made him feel better. In his
second-family life, he was known as having "his own mind," rarely
accepting favors from friends or going along with any group activities *ever!* His off-center stance looked impressive on the surface,
but left him feeling lonely. Frank was a kid who needed to learn to
say, "yes" to other people and to life.

"How Am I Doing?"

Every meeting, 14-year-old Megan would ask to see the latest
sociogram of her second family. As I've mentioned, this is a map of
friends I draw up in the first session, a map that can change radically given the shifting alliances between teens. Megan wanted to
review her sociogram weekly, to see who was "in" and who was
"out." This ritual was a way for Megan to say, "How am I doing this
week?" Since Megan's parents were so in the dark about these
matters, and since no one in her second family could be trusted
with this highly classified information, our relationship became a
witness to her ever-shifting friendships. As Megan became more
secure in herself, she gradually forgot to check out how she was
doing.

GOOD-BYE RITUALS

"Are We on the Same Page?"

With 12-year-old Jen and many other kids, I've developed the same
routine. At the *end* of every session, I ask: "Tell me what you think I
was saying today." Moody, unfocused, multitasking, or language-
disordered teens are not just oppositional. They concretely misun-
derstand what is being said. For example, Jen and I talked about
the difficulty she had inviting classmates over to her house. I sug-

gested that she'd probably have more success if she didn't ask in front of other kids. That's when she'd most likely be turned down. What Jen actually heard me say, however, was "Don't invite any kids to your house. Don't ask at all." What a depressing thought for her, one that almost pushed her out of treatment.

Shawn, a tenth grader, told me he planned to ask out a girl in his class. The two had been friends for a long time; in fact, they'd met in religious school years before. Shawn was going to "pop" the dating question after they left church services. I said, "Great, do it! But, remember, in my experience, it can be tough to change a friendship into a 'dating' relationship." When I asked him to tell me what he thought I was saying, I learned Shawn believed my "it's tough" remark was directed personally at him, as in "You'll never be able to get this girl to go out with you—*someone else probably would.*" Checking it out at the end of the meeting gave me a chance to say "No, I didn't mean just you, I meant it would be tough for anyone. You can ask your uncle. I'll bet he'll tell you the same thing happened to him. And you know what? It happened to me, too."

A brief, good-natured review of what was heard, compared to what was actually said, is an effective ritual, one I often encourage with parents at home. It is a chance to joke around, to correct a message, and to make sure that we are on the same page by the end of the meeting. If kids are going to forget what we've talked about by the time they leave the room, at least it will be what was actually said—a place to begin next time.

"Trash-Talk"

Joey, and numbers of other "slackers," take the garbage out for me every week. At the end of our session, there would be a small bag with leftovers or cellophane wrappers from our snacks. Joey would ask, "You want me to take care of that?" I'd say, "Yeah, sure." We met for a year and a half, and not once did Joey fail to ask if he should take the garbage on his way out.

Again, the ritual had meaning. At home, Joey wasn't expected to do anything except his homework—the one thing, of course, he wouldn't do without a struggle. So, Joey liked our trash ritual. It helped him feel that he had given something back to me, showing his parents and friends he wasn't a total goof-off: "So there!" he seemed to be saying. You can imagine the good-natured ribbing he took from buddies who met him after our meetings, as well as the shock from his perplexed parents.

"Can I Have My Mantra?"

Sixteen-year-old Samantha was referred to me because of anxiety episodes and chronic worrying, which she regulated by wild acting out and pot smoking. At the end of each session, Samantha—a sophisticated, New Age kind of kid—would ask me to give her a "mantra." This would take the form of an affirmation, summing up what we had done during the session. It needed to be something very simple: "This too shall pass." "During the week, smile just once or twice." If I forgot our good-bye ritual, Samantha would immediately remind me: "What's my mantra today?" In the context of her second family of smokers, binge drinkers, and runaways, a simple mantra was like a ring of security to Samantha. Given her three-times-married parents and chaotic first-family configurations, it didn't hurt having a simple memory to ease the constant turmoil all around.

*   *   *

As these examples demonstrate, a ritual is a work of creativity, *interpersonal graffiti*, so to speak—the ritual bears a child's mark. It expresses the uniqueness of the relationship, the comfort and predictability of your space together. It is an anchor in an essentially chaotic life, not nearly predictable enough for the boy or girl you see in your office. It is often a concrete way to open up discussions, almost always leading to troublesome issues in the first family at home or the second family of peers.

Details

Adults in treatment try to get into the details of their lives. After all, grown-ups have *chosen* to be with you, to focus on certain problems, though not necessarily the ones they *need* to focus on. Decades of invisible habits, unconscious motivation, addictions, and rigid character armor bury truth. But at least the choice to work on problems is the client's.

Paradoxically, while teens *see* their issues more clearly than most adults, they *choose* to be secretive with the prying grown-ups who have forced them into treatment. Except in rare cases, the decision to seek help is made by parents, the school, or the court. Your existence in the room is a reminder of a world they cannot control. And, even if a teen is less wary about opening up, they usually haven't developed what school consultant Michael Nerny calls "emotional literacy." Words to describe experiences don't easily come. So, conversation about what really matters may be difficult:

THERAPIST: How did you feel about the weekend?

TEEN: It was OK.

THERAPIST: Didn't you go to that party?

TEEN: Yeah.

THERAPIST: Well, how was it?

TEEN: You know, we hung out and stuff.

Not a pretty picture, but common with teenage clients. We have words to describe the phenomenon: defiance, therapy refusal, selective muteness. But that's about the normal level of detail you're spontaneously going to get. It is nowhere near enough for your client to feel as if you're really in there with him or her—or for you to feel that the material is meaningful to the work.

Of course, the same practically mute adolescent is capable of revealing endless details to friends. In fact, I have come to understand that kids *live* in the details; teens, especially, are obsessed with them. But adults, even child professionals, often consider ordinary *teen* detail to be meaningless. *This is a basic clinical dilemma: it is exactly the kind of endless detail we've been taught to evaluate as defensive that builds a strong connection.* In work with adolescents, the nitty-gritty about what happened is the most direct pathway into a meaningful experience. "I can't believe you're interested in this stuff," one teen after another remarks. I am. *Seemingly trivial, insanely boring details tell me what he is actually doing, thinking, and feeling—and the high-risk decisions that must be made every day.*

Details and Depth

Many clinicians, however, still do not pay attention to trivial details simply for the sake of their content. Typically, we are more interested in what is going on *behind* them: What do they mean? How does the patient feel about them? These are what I call second- or third-level questions. Unfortunately, this traditional line of questioning is practically guaranteed to silence most adolescents, especially when it comes to helping kids develop "emotional literacy"— a voice to describe personal experience and complicated decisions. Since an adolescent lives in the details of life, your endless curiosity and fascination with the trivial *deepens* the relationship. She begins to feel you are seriously interested in *her* story, the "stupid" details that most adults view as a total waste of time.

Here is an example of dialogue that initially focuses on meaningless detail, and ends up opening doors to the most meaningful issues in a teen's life:

THERAPIST: How was the weekend?

AMANDA, A 14-YEAR-OLD: OK. I hung out.

THERAPIST: Who were you with?

AMANDA: Maggie and Alice. Well, Maggie snuck out in this really cool black tank top. Her parents haven't seen it. And Alice wore these new pants, like around her hips, with a big belt.

THERAPIST: What about you? What did you wear? [I restrain myself from moving toward significant issues.]

AMANDA: I had on those new shoes. I have them on today, you want to see them?

Over the next few minutes, Amanda displays her new shoes, and describes their various features—color, the height of the heel, the special laces. Far from being the neutral observer, I comment, reacting to each aspect she points out.

THERAPIST: It sounds like you guys wanted to look pretty good.

AMANDA: Yeah, there's this new girl—I don't know if I told you about her already. Kelly, she's a real bitch. All the guys like her. And, we were going out in a group with her and a bunch of the guys.

THERAPIST: [Again, instead of asking, How do you feel about this new girl, Kelly?, I remain just as deeply grounded in the superficial.] Oh. Who else was there?

AMANDA: You know, Chris, Jake, Matthew, those guys. And Emily was there. Also Devon.

THERAPIST: So, what was everybody else wearing?

AMANDA: Well, just about everybody had on stuff that showed off their tattoos or piercings. Because that's what Kelly's into. She's got a few that her parents don't even have a clue about. Her mom knows about her belly button ring, but Kelly's got her nipple pierced. Her mom has no idea.

THERAPIST: [resisting the temptation to explore the therapeutic gold of mother–daughter relationships, secrets, etc.] So where did you guys go?

AMANDA: We hung out at J.B.'s house.

THERAPIST: What did you do over there?

AMANDA: We smoked up a little. Then a bunch of us went to the tattoo store at the mall, and we talked about the ones we were thinking of getting.

THERAPIST: Which were the best?

AMANDA: Well, there's one I was thinking of. I'd get it on my hip, it's real small, and my mom would never see it. Because even if I was wearing a thong, it couldn't really be seen.

THERAPIST: What does it look like?

AMANDA: It's a little rose. It's like this really beautiful red.

(*Amanda and I talk a bit about the shade of red, how she came to pick that one.*)

AMANDA: But, just when I was almost all ready to do it, I got in a fight with Maggie. She said I was being a poser, and I'm getting a tattoo just because Kelly is now the queen and I'm trying to be like her.

THERAPIST: Well, what are Kelly's piercings and tattoos like?

AMANDA: The big thing is she had her tongue pierced. She was the first one who did that.

THERAPIST: [finally, my first more traditional response] How do you feel about it? Do you think that's a good idea, this tongue piercing?

AMANDA: Well, she can do it, but I'm scared. For her, it's all about hooking up. The boys really like it. But I'm just not ready for that, I don't think, so I'm just going to go for the tattoo instead.

THERAPIST: You're going for the tattoo to look better? So you can find someone to hook up with? Or to pose? Maybe Maggie was right? [finally, a not-so-subtle nudge to think about her motivation] What's the tattoo for?

AMANDA: I don't know. I have to think about that, about what Maggie said. I don't know if I'm just doing it so Kelly will let me in. She's got everybody else. It feels like I don't have the friends I used to.

THERAPIST: Maybe you're right. . . . Who don't you have anymore? Who's gone?

The talk has moved from malls, clothes, and shoes, to tattoos, to "hooking up," to connections with other kids—all the way to abandonment and betrayal. What's really disturbing Amanda is the friends she's lost. Over the next few weeks, this became the core of our work—friends who had moved into a tight circle around Kelly, having left Maggie behind. That is where Amanda really lives. Our discussions could now center on her losses and the decisions she needed to make about creating more secrets from her mother, staying true to herself, whom to connect with, and how to approach them.

BUT, WILL IT WORK WITH BOYS?

Can the same kind of detail-oriented inquiry be used with a boy? I am asked this question in every workshop. We tend to think girls will go into the details, but reticent boys won't. *That is not what I have experienced. If I remain committed to the superficial specifics, boys open up just as readily.*

Eric, 14, was in treatment because of always being "the odd boy out," who would explode at those around. Whether it was religious school, community camps, or classroom politics, Eric never seemed to have a friend. He arrived for a session upset because during the weekend he had been involved in a baseball game that made him furious. He hit a home run that was a game winner. As he rounded third base, a player on the other team made a loud derogatory remark, ruining one of his first moments of "schoolyard glory."

You might think, again, that a useful approach to Eric's terribly discouraging experience would be to ask him "What did you think?"; "How did you feel?"; "What could that whole incident have been about?" These questions would focus on the "presenting problem" of the experience. Instead, here is some of what I asked:

"Was it hot that day?"

"Did the coach say anything to you before going to the plate?"

"What bat did you use?"

"What kind of pitch did you hit?"

"Where did the ball go?"

"Did the kids cheer when you hit the homer, or were they quiet?"

"When you rounded third, what did the other kid say to you?"

"What tone of voice did he use?"

"What was the most insulting thing about what he said?"

"Did you say anything in return?"

"Did any of your friends hear the kid's remark?"

All this led to what really upset Eric, which was not simply that he was put down. It was suburban Little League—with his friends on the team and his parents out in the sidelines, so he felt completely torn between his first and second family. Should he stand up to the kid and diss him back (the second family's choice) or ignore it (his parents' and coach's view)? He chose the latter approach and said nothing.

Worse, after the game a number of kids went over to a teammate's house without telling Eric. He didn't know why; once again, he hadn't been included. Eric assumed it was because he'd been such a "wuss"; he wanted to ask one of those kids to come over to his house for a sleepover but, extremely shy to begin with, Eric had no idea how, especially after the incident at the game.

The session moved from a description of which bat Eric chose, to the details of his hit, to the incident itself, to the dilemma about the right thing to do, to defining himself as a "loser," to maintaining the connection with his friends, to feeling left out and not having a clue as to how to move on.

*   *   *

Details tell the story. For teens, stories about trivial matters almost always lead to real-life decisions. Since a lot of what happens with adolescents are first-time experiences, they must make many decisions about whether to involve themselves in high-risk behaviors. Talking about the details helps them tell the story in a way that is alive. Emotional literacy builds a foundation for talking about tough decisions with another person. These details are the soil of the work. They allow the relationship to grow—if you are willing to fully engage with them.

Full-Frontal Engagement

Full engagement intensifies the relationship; it solidifies the connection between adult and adolescent. By full-frontal engagement I
mean:

♦ The small details that matter to kids, matter to you.

♦ Your reactions are not delivered from a slightly removed,
  "neutral" place.

♦ Your values-based experiences in life, your "adult" reactions,
  are not to be hidden; they are part and parcel of the exchange.

♦ You express yourself with heartfelt, real feeling.

♦ Your reactions to specific events, as well as to life values, are
  made absolutely clear.

♦ You are willing to "mix it up" with kids over differences of
  opinion.

♦ You are selectively open about your feelings of frustration,
  pride, outrage, and worry—those reactions adolescents regularly provoke.

Full-frontal engagement is essential to building a therapeutic
relationship with teens, and it differs markedly from traditional
models of therapy.

HEY DUDE, WHERE'S MY SHRINK?

For several reasons, most therapy models, which remove the therapist in subtle but significant ways, do not work with teens. Lots of
questions—without opinion, debate, sympathy, disagreement, and
advice—put kids to sleep. And, too much technique often shuts
them up. Not coincidentally, post-World War II parents have been
offered four decades of technique-oriented childrearing prescrip-
tions. Parents: Do not impose your reactions. Kids must find their

own answers. Build a welcoming, safe space, and they will come. Try this wholesale technique and they will respond.

Unfortunately, hanging back ever so slightly, asking too many questions about feelings, and using linear techniques feels one-dimensional to many adolescents. *These approaches do not create traction, a vital edge of relatedness between therapist and client; they do not help an adolescent feel you are really there, in a three-dimensional way.* Contemporary kids are used to the opposite in their everyday lives—on-going repartee with friends, cyber-space dialogue, and interactive TV. Listen to the dialogue that typically goes on between a teen and his peers. You will surely notice a back and forth, an in-the-moment, mixing-it-up exchange that is all about the edgy, edge of relatedness.

It is hard for helping professionals to move beyond what we have been trained to do. But with adolescents, full engagement is absolutely necessary. It creates a relationship that is compelling to a teen, perhaps the only engaged experience with a grown-up in his or her life.

Smoking Up

Sixteen-year-old Simon and I talked a little about what he had been up to over the previous week, Simon mentioned, almost in passing, that he and a couple of friends had smoked pot in the bathroom at school. The conversation continued as follows.

THERAPIST: You smoked up in the bathroom? Are you insane?! [His school's policy of immediate expulsion was well known. I was shocked he'd been so brazen and I wasn't going to hide it.]

SIMON: What? Dr. Taffel, you don't get it. No way we could have gotten caught.

THERAPIST: Yeah, right. What are the doors like, are they sealed?

SIMON: Real tight, it's the teacher's bathroom. We thought of that.

THERAPIST: Nobody comes in afterwards? You thought about that, too, I suppose?

SIMON: No. It was the last period of the day. No one's around. [Simon had all the bases covered!] I'm telling you, we were on top of it.

THERAPIST: You're driving me up the wall! What if you *did* get caught? Let's say someone unexpectedly walked in.

SIMON: (*after thinking for a minute*) Kids use the teacher's bathroom more than teachers. But what are the chances another kid would rat us out?

THERAPIST: Well, you're right, probably not much. [Full-engagement must be based on assessing the truth in what kids are saying.] But, how about the cafeteria cook? He could have smelled the smoke.

SIMON: That guy is really cool.

THERAPIST: The cook? What's he got to do with this?

SIMON: Well, we all go to him for advice. He's got the best perspective in that whole place. He says, like, when you're a teenager, that's when kids are supposed to have fun. He tells us not to get crazy about any one girl. [Simon was having trouble with his girlfriend around this time.] He gives better advice than the guidance counselor. No offense, sometimes better than you.

This exchange led right into the *real* issue on Simon's mind: He was angry about the lack of good advice from supposedly informed adults, including me. In turn, we talked about taking risks with pot and then, in detail, about what to do with his girlfriend. For several meetings, we spoke about moving from the early adolescent boy world of goofing off and screwing around to decisions regarding his first real love experience with a girl.

Gritty Nitty-Gritty Details

Here is a more hardcore example of "engagement"—without commentary—so its rawness can be directly experienced.

SHAWNA [age 15, who lives in an affluent suburb]: (*midway through a session*) This really cute guy is going to convince me to do it with him. I know it. I can feel it.

THERAPIST: Have you been hooking up with him already?

SHAWNA: Yeah.

THERAPIST: What have you done so far?

SHAWNA: Well, at this party in another town everyone was getting pretty wasted. I flashed him and we got together later.

THERAPIST: Where did you go?

SHAWNA: We ditched everybody and went to his younger brother's room.

THERAPIST: Where? What was his room like?

SHAWNA: They're so rich, but it was kind of cramped and smelly. But we really started to hook up. He's such a great kisser.

THERAPIST: What makes him so great?

SHAWNA: It's not sloppy but it's really deep. And it just turns me on. We made out for hours. Then I went down on him. He talked to me about it for a long time while we were in there, and I just decided to do it.

THERAPIST: Oh, no, you didn't! You just met this guy and you just went down on him?

SHAWNA: Well, I knew him from being around before. He's one of the hot boys. Everybody's had their eye on him for a long time. I was the first.

THERAPIST: OK, he's hot. But I still can't believe you did this after meeting him for a few minutes.

SHAWNA: We were kind of wasted. I didn't want to stop. And I'm gonna tell you, it was great.

THERAPIST: What about going down?

SHAWNA: Well, that's the one thing. It's kind of graphic. Are you going to get all grossed out about this?

THERAPIST: Maybe. I don't know.

SHAWNA: I mean, you have a daughter around my age. Doesn't it really freak you out to hear this?

THERAPIST: Yeah, actually it does. And I'm not exactly sure I want all the details. But tell you what, I'll let you know if I get scared or too embarrassed.

SHAWNA: It was the position. He wanted to be on top. He wanted to come on my face. Like with a lot of boys, that's really important to him; he had to be on top of me. And, someone could have opened the door.

THERAPIST: How long did he have to be on top of you?

SHAWNA: It took forever. And being under him all that time was kind of weird. It was like, I was less than him.

THERAPIST: Well, you really were. I feel bad about that.

SHAWNA: Yeah. I couldn't move my head. I mean, I guess it was fun. I won't lie. But, something about the whole thing. . . . I felt smaller than I felt before. Here I got this guy that everybody thinks is so hot. But I felt smaller. And, I think that's why I've been fighting with everybody this week.

Our uncomfortable exchange led to Shawna's sense of self-worth (the first time we had gotten into that area), what being a girl meant to her, whether she wanted to hook up with this boy *for herself* or how much was it really about beating out the other girls.

*   *   *

Your natural reactions, informed by hard-won experience as an adult, are not to be kept out of the room. Adult responsiveness is what makes the exchange come alive. It motivates and nurtures real engagement. Of course, your reactions must be tempered to fit the child across from you and open to continuous reflection. Most of us know the parameters of careful self-reflection and attunement. We are stunted, however, when it comes to the kind of responsiveness that teens get from each other and secretly wish from adults.

Sometimes it is the spontaneity of the reaction that makes it uniquely effective.

Full engagement shows adolescents that you are actually listening. If you do not respond fully, you will probably get half the story. Most teens would be convinced, and correctly so, that you are yet another adult who is too programmed, too held-in to be moved by what is really important.

Full engagement loosens teens up. Without planning to, kids do the unthinkable—begin telling you more about what actually happened. Again, details lead not only to a fuller story, but to nitty-gritty decisions about what to do today, tomorrow, and in the future. With Simon, that decision was whether he was going to smoke up again in school or move on to a real relationship with his girlfriend. Shawna needed to decide how (and whether) to be in charge of her sexuality, at the next party and every weekend after that.

*   *   *

Kids in helping relationships with adults need a full partner. They live their lives with few adults who will engage them in trivial details, which leads an exciting and hopeful thought. Therapists who are fully engaged are in a position to begin healing the "divided self" of 21st-century teens.

THE CORE

Healing the Divided Self of 21st-Century Teens

One thing you can't hide is when you're crippled inside.
—*John Lennon, "Crippled Inside"*

TV ruined my imagination and my ability to . . . um . . . um . . . um . . . well, you know.
—*Bart Simpson*

Now that basic parameters of the relationship have been established, a significant part of working with today's adolescents involves challenging them to deepen. Any successful helping relationship must question unhealthy aspects of teen life that are considered normal by cultural myths. Kids are short changed if we quietly accept beliefs about adolescence that stunt their development and potential for greater resilience. With this in mind:

I challenge kids to talk more to their parents—about the things that actually matter.

I challenge kids to be more empathic and open their hearts—to consider their impact on parents, teachers, and friends.

I challenge adolescents to become good at something—to develop an unselfconscious passion.

Why is challenge in these three areas—emotional expressiveness, empathy toward others and the development of passion—such a central part of treating teens? Because so much of kids' life is focused on external packaging, rather than on building a strong core self.

The Divided Self in Post-Victorian Times

Adolescents do not just experience a split between the first family at home and the second family out there, they live with an internal, psychic split as well. The "divided self" was a widely held clinical theory for decades, and it has profound relevance for today's teens. Clinicians such as Melanie Klein (*The Psychoanalysis of Children*, 1949), Margaret Mahler (*The Psychological Birth of the Human Infant*, 1975), Michael Balint (*The Basic Fault*, 1968), and R. D. Laing (*The Divided Self*, 1969) described a normal psychic split in the development of very young children. In this "paranoid–schizoid" position, which Klein postulated arising within the first year, the self is organized around ruthless greed, a sense that the world is vindictive, and a lack of empathy or guilt about one's impact on others. The continuation of a split self into adulthood was thought to be the result of various kinds of insufficient early mothering. Treatment could be a curative experience in which the self was unified, with clients moving further along the developmental continuum into "the depressive position."

Though certainly not inviting at first glance, the depressive position is a true accomplishment. It is the ability to form deep relationships and the capacity to handle ambivalence, that is, to "hold" both love and hate. It is the uncomfortable experience of guilt when wrong is done. It is the emotional wisdom that relationships require empathy toward others. Work and creativity are now more possible, because expression of one's true self allows for genuine desire and uninhibited passion.

The Divided Self in 21st-Century Adolescents

Most teens, thankfully, do not suffer from the kind of early maternal deprivation these writers describe. In fact, a lot of what our psychological pioneers hypothesized is now understood to be constitutional—not the fault of archetypical "bad mothering." However, many kids who end up in our offices do suffer from what I call a *culturally induced divided self.* The very existence of this divided state is part of their ordinary lives and, therefore, almost invisible. This is so because kids are challenged in all the wrong ways, endlessly pushed into developing a weaker sense of self.

From very early on, they are challenged to cultivate a veneer—to dress right, to get the right stuff, and to become voracious consumers. They are seduced into worshipping physical perfection, to strive for an absolutely flawless body. They are slowly encouraged not to talk about internal experience, but rather to be glibly articulate, to diss, or to dispense the hollow wisdom of mass-market psychobabble. They are challenged by national testing to measure up on standardized tests—from preschool through to high school—often without understanding the material and without a love of learning.

They are clearly instructed to maintain a "wall of silence," not to approach adults until a friend is practically drowning. They are challenged to multitask, to engage in as many activities as possible, without necessarily mastering one passion deeply. More and more are challenged to develop a meaningless "résumé" for college, to sign up for extracurricular activities and community service points because it is expected of them, not because of inner commitment.

Kids are challenged to create portable relationships: to develop superficial connections with professional grown-ups—coaches, after-school leaders, tutors, program directors, religious instructors and social-skill facilitators. Some do challenge, but their coming and going is structured into the assembly line of normal development. Kids move along a virtual conveyor belt from one child wrangler to the next. It is almost impossible for any adult to *mentor,* to be around long enough to encourage kids to put off instant gratification or to handle the frustration necessary to achieve mastery.

Do Mental Health Professionals Challenge Kids?

Enter therapists into this mass production of false-self experience. Unfortunately, many traditional forms of treatment do not sufficiently challenge, either. Younger clients can play for months or even years at a time, while the therapy provides a supportive environment. Therapeutic inquiry or interpretation does not easily move teens over hurdles to embrace passion, parents, or even friendship. In a special-effects world, traditional therapeutic interventions are quickly overshadowed by the next video game, the next dramatic e-mail or the next second-family fling. No wonder the newer end of the therapeutic continuum is so appealing. Kids may be temporarily challenged by recent approaches: cognitive-behavioral therapy, dialectic behavioral therapy, posttrauma protocols, antibully programs, and social-emotional learning modules, to name just a few. Such techniques are invaluable, but when primarily offered to the most disturbed clients in an impersonal, short-term package (as is often the case), kids are not stretched to dig deep, reason differently and heal internal, emotional splits.

Treatment, as I propose it, ought not to mirror the fragmented nature of our world. It must challenge a significant number of kids before it is too late, precisely because they are not being challenged in their 21st-century lives. Challenged in all the wrong ways, teens end up feeling trapped in a "paranoid–schizoid position." They are poseurs fearful that they will be revealed. They live in a world that often mocks kids who demonstrate true passion, that is disdainful of genuine empathy, and that discourages relationships with responsible adults—all necessary for the development of a strong core self.

Through the challenge of relationship with you, teens may turn more to their parents. They may not be quite so ashamed of their real feelings. They may develop un-self-conscious passion. They may become capable of more compassion toward friends and lovers. In other words, through challenge, kids' divided self may heal just enough to help them get healthier.

Talking More to Parents

One of my central goals is to help teens stop believing that parents or other responsible adults can never understand, that real talk is reserved only for other kids. This is a culturally reinforced notion child professionals need to challenge. *I hope teens will talk more to their parents—so that they will need to talk less to me.* The principle behind this challenge is fairly obvious: The less a child talks about what is actually going on in his life, the further he moves away from the first family at home and toward the second family. Out there, kids begin engaging in riskier behaviors, the very activities that make them uneasy about opening up enough to feel connected to adults. Even after a few weeks of this cycle, parents have almost no idea about what is going on with their kids, and are less able to intelligently guide them.

Of course, normal differentiation comes with the turf of teen years, but these days psychic distance begins much earlier. By fourth or fifth grades (rather than junior high school), many kids *naturally* drift from their mothers and fathers toward the parallel universe of the second family. They know that secrets must be kept behind the wall of silence. Even good kids understand "the rules," and competent parents are left in the dark. The entire culture believes this state of affairs is normal, despite its beginning in mid-elementary school. The creation of "tweens," a newly coined developmental term, normalizes this earlier shift toward adolescent behavior: "My 10-year-old daughter's becoming an adolescent, that's why she doesn't talk. I don't really expect her to say much to me." From even younger children: "I have my friends. What kid my age talks to adults?"

CHALLENGE THE MYTH THAT KIDS NEVER TALK

After decades working with adolescents, I have come to understand that this is a destructive, self-perpetuating myth. *Teens do talk.* Unfortunately, they talk at all the "wrong" times—when they want something, when they're scared, when they're negotiating, and when parents are distracted. It is an equally inaccurate myth that boys, in particular, do not talk. I've spoken with thousands of families and have learned that boys are not simply junior versions of "withholding" men. Many boys these days talk to their parents (even mothers), throughout the adolescent years, and girls, counter to stereotype, may be less revealing than the myth allows. Countless mothers have said to me, "I thought that my daughter would be more open. I expected in these modern times we'd have that close mother–daughter relationship. My son has been no more secretive about what's actually going on."

Why? Girls are catching up to boys in terms of risky second-family behavior. The latest national studies found teenage girls to be engaging in substances and sexuality at rates almost as early and frequently as boys ("2003 Youth High Risk Behavior Survey," Grunbaum, Kann, Kinchen, et al.). Girls also feel trapped into peer secretiveness about what friends tell them. They, too, live behind a wall of silence, knowing full well the price to be paid by any teen who reveals another's issues. Therefore boys *and* girls may clam up on schedule at 12 or 13, not just because of "developmentally appropriate differentiation." More often than adults realize it's because he or she is afraid to inadvertently let slip that a friend has an eating disorder, another has had casual sex, another has been cutting school or cutting herself. It was a real discovery when I finally understood that many kids stop talking to parents not because they want to, but because they are afraid of putting their friends at risk.

At the same time, most adolescents feel that they are *supposed* to be uncommunicative to parents. Hundreds of TV shows written by kids (well, 20-something adults—or younger) just *for* kids create worlds in which parents are irrelevant; they seem not to exist. Programs like *7th Heaven, The O.C.,* and *American Dreams* made an impression precisely because they've gone against cultural myths, introducing the possibility that some teens really do talk to parents. But these are notable precisely because they are exceptions.

Powerful everyday forces make it essential to challenge the perceived and real communication chasm before your teen client and his or her parents drift even further away from each other.

ASK THE UNASKABLE

A major part of a child professional's job is to reverse this cycle. More talking leads to greater mutual understanding; real information helps parents better guide kids; informed advice leads to greater trust. The cycle can be reversed—*if* we challenge the notion that teen silence at home is normal.

In private sessions, I question kids' assumptions that they cannot talk to their parents. I repeat this message to parents: "The distance between you and your adolescent is not as inevitable as you think." *I regularly pose unaskable questions.* I demonstrate my belief that kids and parents can actually talk together about almost anything. My iconoclastic curiosity is informed by Harry Stack Sullivan's interpersonal school of psychoanalysis, in which "the inquiry" itself leads to an expansion of what clients believe is possible. When challenging kids about what they take for granted—clamming up at home says that *nothing is off limits.* Questioning their reluctance to discuss the undiscussable—second-family activities, sex, drugs, eating, love, and so on—throws kids off-guard. Sixteen-year-old Lilianna asked me point-blank: "Why do you think it's so important to talk to my mother; no one expects this from a kid my *age!*" "That's the problem," I replied. "No one does expect it, and you're worse off—more anxious and more alone— because of this belief. Give it time, you'll see what I mean." Interestingly, Lilianna's parents had a similar reaction: "You really believe she'll talk to us? That's why we sent her to you!" My response, "Exactly. One of my main goals is to help her be more open with you, not just me. I'll help you deal with it."

Following are a few ordinary and some of the more outrageous areas I encourage kids to talk about with the adults at home:

Douglas mentioned to me his plans to have sex with an older girl he'd been hanging out with. I asked: "Have you told your parents you're considering sex with Matty? What do you think your mother's reaction is going to be? Maybe your father will have more understanding about this than you give him credit for. Or maybe they won't, we don't know yet."

Jordan was viciously scapegoated in school and felt miserable about it. Over time, he became more and more embarrassed about bringing this up to his parents. The sullen distance that developed led to hurt feelings on his dad's part, which increasingly erupted into battles over unrelated issues. Whenever Jordan told me about yet another new bullying incident, I asked: "Did you mention it at home? Did you tell your dad?"

Millie's body had changed dramatically. Going to the mall became a dreaded event, given all the head turning and advances she had to deal with. I regularly asked Millie, "Did you bring this up with your mother? What do you think her reaction would be?" Why don't you think she'd understand?"

Sophie told me about hanging out at Zoe's house with no adult supervision, as well as her concerns about a close friend's health. I said: "Do you mention to your mom you have this bad feeling that Zoe is bulimic and throwing up every day?"

These questions seem absurd to ask an adolescent. Frankly, the initial response is often, "No way!" or "Are you crazy?" If the therapist is a "bridge" though, kids' and parents' disbelief is worth challenging. When I asked 16-year-old Douglas if he could talk to his mom about plans to have sex with his girlfriend, Douglas said: "Are you insane? My mom preaches affirmations from the Bible. How in the world am I going to say stuff to her about sex?"

Sophie's first response was "If I tell her that Zoe is bulimic, my mom would get so crazed she'd call up Zoe's mother up right away. I'd lose Zoe as a friend. And everyone would hate me."

Likewise, Jordan's first reaction was to become furious that I would suggest that he reveal to Dad what an outcast he was.

ASKING CREATES CHANGE

♦ *Asking detoxifies poisonous myths.* It diminishes a teenager's inability to even *imagine* that such talk could happen. For example, besides becoming sexually active, Douglas also was involved in writing graffiti. I asked him regularly about his various friends, how they snuck out to write, and *why he never mentioned it to his parents.* I brought it up in so many ways that the subject eventually became normalized. One day Douglas casually mentioned graffiti during a phone call with his father. Douglas asked what Dad felt about graffiti around town, whether it added or detracted from the urban scene. From that minidiscussion, the boy finally got around to admitting to his parents that he had been a "writer" for some time and that, by the way, he was no longer a virgin, either. There were some temporary fireworks between them, but it represented the first constructive dialogue about real issues for years.

♦ *Kids' responses say a lot about family dances at home.* As stuck interactions become more apparent, you learn what needs to be worked on.

I repeatedly asked Jordan why he would not reveal the extent of the abuse he endured at school. After a while, I understood that it was impossible for him to talk to his dad, Evan, during the week. In the midst of frenetic schedules and worries about professional issues, Evan was always on edge. It was far better to approach him on the weekends when he felt less the "alpha" male. He might then be able to grasp some of the torture Jordan was experiencing, without becoming impatient about his son's lack of popularity or assertiveness.

♦ *Better advice may come from parents than one can possibly imagine.* Even expressing the *possibility* of change helps some kids shift their thinking about parents and, in turn, themselves.

Fourteen-year-old Amanda had been going past her "safety zone" drinking. Just about every time she would tell me about weekend bashes, I'd ask, "Have you discussed this with your mother?" And, almost every time, Amanda would remind me about the "craziness of this request" and would patronizingly ignore the question. "It will make you less anxious, hiding less," I insisted. Meanwhile, her grades and relationships with friends were tanking, as was her confidence. Finally, one night at 3:00 in the morning, Amanda was so nauseated from shots of tequila, she couldn't sleep. Neither could her mom. The two inadvertently bumped into each other, sat down over the kitchen table and had one of those open talks about drinking reserved for the last 30 seconds of teen TV. Amanda was stunned; her mother was shaken, but Amanda's anxiety significantly lessened. A week later she told me how much older she felt at home. This confidence translated into slightly less drinking and considerably more independence from her second-family friends.

A secret graffiti writer, a loser, and a drinker—talking about true-self experience with parents. This heals some of the emotional split within teenagers. They become less withdrawn and paranoid about adults discovering who they really are. Your challenge initiates a struggle between personal secrets and the wall of silence.

Empathizing More with Parents

Teens need to understand who their parents are. Emphasizing empathy toward mothers and fathers represents a reversal from the mantra of post-World War II childrearing: *Parents must try to understand their children.* D. W. Winnicott believed that empathy toward parents, moving beyond blame of one's parents for disappointments, errors, neglect, and so on, was a sign of growing maturity. A more complex view of their humanity marked a stronger sense of self, signaling that the analysis was nearing termination.

The psychological establishment has begun to move "back to the future," toward Winnicott's wisdom. But this is mostly in a horizontal direction. Schools focus on peer-to-peer empathy—a major component of antibully programs and social-emotional intelligence. The idea, however, that *empathy begins at home, toward parents,* is still largely ignored. Parents are presented to kids—by the media, by each other, and by therapists—as being two-dimensional. There isn't much value placed on understanding parents except as someone to blame (mental health professionals) or as a means to an end (culture and kids)—for more money, a later curfew, an empty house. Empathy toward kids was a necessary reaction to repressive homes in which children "were seen but not heard." And, while parental empathy helps kids escape some pathology, a pendulum swing in the absolute opposite direction does little good. Parents as two-dimensional stick figures who are without feelings further divide 21st-century teens. Kids feel mean, out of control, and out of touch with their hurtful impact on their most significant adults.

The relationship with you is an opportunity to create an

empathic challenge: *The more adolescents are able to grasp who their parents are, the more they can recognize the impact of their own behavior on others.* Empathic connections at home translate into greater awareness in the peer group and with adults. It is a step toward healing an adolescent's divided self. When you ask a teen to *know* when she's being mean toward Mom or Dad, she actually has a chance to do something about it.

PARENTS ARE PEOPLE TOO

When Samantha says her mother, Harriet, goes out of her mind if she ever tells her anything about her private life, she's right. Because I know Harriet, I understand how Mom worries about the nefarious adolescent world. However, I also see what Sam can't see. Harriet gets so upset because both her parents died suddenly and she cannot tolerate being taken by surprise. If Sam's provocative, last-minute announcements could be handled differently, Mom might not respond in such a "crazy" way—quite a challenge to this relentlessly impatient teenage girl.

Sean cannot picture saying anything to his father, Pete, about personal relationships, because Dad begins lecturing. He tells Sean exactly what he *ought* to do and takes a condescending tone toward him. What Sean doesn't understand is that he speaks to his father in such an insulting way, Pete experiences constant *hurt*. Instead of saying he is hurt (because "a father" isn't supposed to show such emotions), Pete sounds gruff. Understandably, Sean has a hard time realizing that "furious" dad is really "hurt" dad. My job is to help Sean get the impact of his words on his father. Of course, Sean thinks I am way out of line to suggest that empathy toward parents is any of his concern. Sean only wants *his* experience understood. I'm more than willing to struggle for this—but not without challenging Sean to look at himself.

When 14-year-old Kyle says he can't talk about a later curfew without his parents flying off the handle, he's also right. Kyle's mother and father *are* overly protective. They get unbelievably anxious about his adolescent comings and goings. It's also true that Kyle demands his curfew be lifted in such a whiny, babyish way, it makes them more convinced he can't handle the temptations that come with staying out later. Because of their dangerous experiences growing up, both having been victims of street violence, Kyle's babyish tone is like chalk on a blackboard. Kyle's challenge is to see the impact whining has on his chronically traumaticized parents.

PUSH KIDS BEYOND STEREOTYPES ABOUT PARENTS

I don't want to hear complaints about parents that are vague or stereotypical. If a teen talks about how his parents are not fair, how they treat his brother better than him, I need to hear just what they're not being fair about. When kids say their parents are "annoying" simply because they're parents, I want to know exactly what they are doing wrong. When a teenager says her parents are "the only ones who won't allow . . . ," I want details. Vague, culturally reinforced stereotypes thwart the development of empathy across the generational divide. We do not normally think of parents as being the victims of abuse, but when it comes to being understood by teens, they often are.

Over time, I want kids to do *more* of the impossible, *to think from both sides of the equation*. I ask kids to envision ahead of time how they might handle interactions with parents and friends differently—given who they are and how they come across. The research of Myrna Shure, author of *Raising a Thinking Child* (1994), has been particularly valuable in this aspect of working with teens. Shure developed a methodology—for children ages three and up—to think about interpersonal situations and how they might handle matters in the future. If a child had a problem on a playdate or sharing in school, he is encouraged to come up with ideas about approaching the playdate or the sharing problem differently the next time. Shure's methodology is used with kids of all ages across the country. Thousands of children have by now been followed to see whether the intervention had any long-term impact. It has been demonstrated that those taught to empathically problem-solve from an early age are better able to deal with interpersonal difficulties, even as they get older.

Informed by Shure's approach, I want *teens* to think about what they can do differently. I challenge them to see their own behavior, empathize with the other's experience, and, then, determine how to solve the issue. As will be apparent, I try to be "vigorously honest" (to quote that guru of parenting—Ozzy Osbourne).

In the following examples, I had been meeting with parents, so I knew a great deal about their beliefs and their inner experiences. Being an empathic bridge challenges the status quo, the divide that splits teens internally from their better selves and interpersonally from their parents.

Kyle is the whiny 14-year-old who complained that his curfew wasn't late enough. The specific issue on Kyle's mind was his desperate need to go to a rock concert the following Friday.

KYLE: I've got it all planned out. I'll get my father just when he comes home from work. He hasn't talked to my mother yet. Then I'll talk to her after dinner, after I get an answer from my father.

THERAPIST: Do you think your mother is going to like being ganged-up on?

KYLE: Ha . . . OK, I'll talk to her first, when she's cooking. She's always in a good mood then.

THERAPIST: What will you say to her?

KYLE: That everybody's going, that I have to go. See, I don't want to make it a choice for her, but I'll just get her thinking about what time it should be and how I'll get there and stuff like that. It's a method called distraction. I learned it watching Court TV.

THERAPIST: So, you're not asking permission from either of them. Do your mom and dad strike you as the type who like being told what they have to do?

KYLE: Are you kidding? They never like to be ordered around. You ought to see my dad when he's being hassled in his business. . . . So, what's your point?

THERAPIST: That you're ordering them into this concert idea. I don't mean this critically, but—it's a ridiculous approach. Knowing your parents as well as I do, it is going to go absolutely nowhere. You're ignoring who they are.

KYLE: OK, so I'll try this instead. I'll blackmail them—like, if you don't let me go, I won't do anything around the house anymore.

THERAPIST: Now you sound like a three-year-old. Do you really want to go to this concert? Because, no offense intended, these approaches are pretty babyish. Why should your parents allow you such a grown-up privilege?

At this point there is a long pause. Kyle is angry.

KYLE: Maybe I'll talk to them together. Maybe I *do* need their permission.

THERAPIST: Well, are you going to talk to them about who else is going?

KYLE: (*whining*) Do they have to know everything? I don't want them to start calling up everybody else.

THERAPIST: Then earn their trust. Make it so they don't feel worried enough that they have to call everybody. You're right, I know they worry a lot. You're going to have to learn how to handle that.

KYLE: Can't you do this for me?

THERAPIST: Hey, I'm not your agent. Anyway, I don't have to live with them, and the truth is you do. So you're the one who has to earn it.

KYLE: I won't go into details, but I'll just ask their permission. It is my first concert, so I'll make it an early curfew, like 2:00 A.M.

THERAPIST: I'm glad you don't have to negotiate anything for me, because I can't believe how bad you are at this. Do you really think 2:00 A.M. is something they're going to agree to for the first time? Remember, they do tend to worry.

KYLE: It's just a beginning; it's what they call a starting point in negotiating.

THERAPIST: But you're going to make them so nervous that it will only backfire on you.

KYLE: (*after another long pause*) So, you think that's too late. But the concert only gets started around 10:00.

THERAPIST: It's your first concert. You know your parents.

KYLE: Maybe 12:00 or 12:30, that doesn't sound so bad. I'll see how they react. And I'll promise that I'll call them.

THERAPIST: Now you're thinking. Is there anything else you're going to promise them? A lot goes on at a concert, and, like most worriers, they're pretty good at imagining the worst.

KYLE: I think that's enough.

THERAPIST: Hmmm. I'm not sure. What about the all the smoking and drinking? You know what happens at concerts.

KYLE: I can't promise not to try if something is passed to me.

THERAPIST: I guess I know where I'll find you Friday night—at home. That's where you'll be.

KYLE: So, what you're saying is I have to promise them not to do anything?

THERAPIST: It's your call. Just remember who your parents are.

What happened after that? Kyle talked to his parents together. They flipped out, just as he had predicted. At first, he couldn't help but whine, couldn't help but come up with the really late curfew, figuring that would be a better bargaining strategy. As if on cue, they threatened to call the other parents. But after a while, Kyle's tone softened and his parents started to settle down. The atmosphere changed dramatically when he said that since this was his first concert, he would only stay until 11:30, go with a friend his parents knew, and have his parents pick him up afterward. Feeling taken into account, they agreed. *After a rocky start, Kyle found a more empathic voice that could be heard by his parents.*

*   *   *

Fifteen-year-old Millie was thinking about whether or not she would have oral sex with the boy she'd been seeing. Her mother, of course, didn't know this, and neither did she know that Millie had already been sexually active, casually hooking up with both boys and girls at weekend parties. Millie and I had talked about various aspects of sex, and I asked if she had ever mentioned any of this to her mother.

> MILLIE: Are you crazy? Would your daughter say anything to you? Would you want her to?
>
> THERAPIST: Your mother is a lot cooler than I am; she's not such a worrier.
>
> MILLIE: No, no, you're wrong, she's completely hysterical about this stuff. Which is really stupid. Wasn't she wild when she was young? But I can't talk about this hardcore stuff. She still thinks I'm making out and just with boys.
>
> THERAPIST: Yeah, but you have this really big decision you've got to make now, about having oral sex or going even further—and I think that she'll be able to help.
>
> MILLIE: How in the world could she be objective?
>
> THERAPIST: You're right, I don't think she could be objective, at first. But then she'll calm down, and maybe she'll give you better advice, as an experienced woman, than I can as a man.
>
> MILLIE: This is insane! I could talk to my mother about giving some boy head? She thinks I'm still a little girl.
>
> THERAPIST: Do you really think she's that stupid? What about the way you dress? Do you think she hasn't noticed? What about the fact that your thong sticks out and you pur-

posely wear it that way? And your tank tops? You don't think she's getting the idea? She's talked to me about the way guys, and in fact girls, too, stare at you in the mall.

MILLIE: (*after a very long pause*) Well, we talk about the sex scenes on TV. We talk about this one being hot and that one not being hot. But she can't know anything about what's happening with me.

THERAPIST: Look at your mother. Take a good look at her. She's beautiful. And you're right, she was pretty wild as a kid. You know what, maybe you've been watching too much TV. She's more like the Osbournes than Ozzie and Harriet.

MILLIE: (*after thinking this over for a minute*) I don't even know how I'd bring it up.

THERAPIST: Just be direct. Maybe it's exactly what's on her mind about you anyway. She might get nervous, but she might also be relieved. I don't know. Just look at her— think about it till next week. Something has to break soon, because she has to know that things are changing.

What happened next? Millie couldn't talk to her mother, Joan, directly. Instead, she left an e-mail in the printer that included a lot of graphic information, and her mother "accidentally" came across it. At first, Mom was a little hysterical. Then she and Millie started talking. Millie began telling her not about sex per se, but about how much she'd been obsessing about her body. This got Joan's sympathy, because she'd felt oppressed by many of the same issues: changing bodies, how you can't be too thin, all the competition. Millie then began to mention other girls she knew and how many of them had had sex, much more extensively than her mother realized. Then they talked about oral sex as a way of having sex that wasn't as embarrassing, because with your clothes on, the boy didn't have to see your body.

This was a huge conversation for them. It led to other conversations, in which Millie actually talked to Joan about having been with a girl. She (like a surprising number of 21st-century mothers I've spoken to) preferred Millie experiment initially with a girl, because at least it was safer than sex with a boy. Joan was, indeed, jangled about all this information, but far less worried about what was going on with Millie, and even more amazed that this conversation had even been possible. Her daughter was beginning to talk to her.

* * *

Walker, in his sophomore year of high school, had been accepted into an excellent after-school training program, and he wanted to get his father to pay some part of the expenses that were looming. Walker's parents were divorced, his dad was very controlling about money, and Walker was extremely resentful about that. He had seen his older brother have terrible arguments until he finally squeezed tiny amounts of money from their father. Walker wanted to be different, but he couldn't imagine how to get started. We practiced, focusing not just on Walker's experiences but also his estranged dad's.

WALKER: My mother wants to confront him herself, but I think I need to.

THERAPIST: How would you bring it up?

WALKER: I'll tell him, "You owe my mother."

THERAPIST: Well, that's not a great start. You know your dad. I've met him several times. Isn't he still angry at your mother? I mean, how would he respond to that?

WALKER: I don't care. I want him to know he hasn't lived up to his end of the bargain.

THERAPIST: Knowing something about your father's experience, I think you need to try another approach.

WALKER: I'll make it real different. I'll say, "You know, Dad, Mom works really hard, and she deserves to have less trouble."

THERAPIST: Still, even though that's how you feel, think about how that puts you right in the middle between them. What's most important to you?

WALKER: I want the money, but I want him to admit that he's been fucking off, too.

THERAPIST: I understand. But I think you're going to have to make up your mind—whether to offend him or whether to be effective.

WALKER: But, I'll sound mad anyway, because that's how I feel.

THERAPIST: I know you feel that way, I really do. But, given the legal history, if you want help, you're going to have to do it in a way that doesn't sound like you're a lawyer representing your mother.

WALKER: (*after thinking for a while*) I'll say, "OK, Dad, I got into this good program; you know it costs a lot of money. What do you think about it?"

THERAPIST: Now, you're being too vague. It's better, but since he's very practical, I think he won't get what you're driving at.

WALKER: I guess I could call him and say, "Dad, we just got the bill. The program costs a lot of money. I'd like you to add as much as you can. What can you do?"

THERAPIST: That sounds a lot better to me. I imagine he'll be less angry. I don't know what he'll do, but knowing him, my guess is that he'll slow things down a little. So, you need to be prepared. How would you feel if he did make an excuse—how would you handle it if he slowed things down?

WALKER: I don't know.

Walker didn't say anything to his father for a couple of weeks. Finally, he brought the subject up in the way he'd practiced with me, and his father's response was to ask for a copy of the training course materials. Ordinarily, if Walker hadn't been prepared, he would have become absolutely furious. But he told me, "I didn't get that mad. And I could see for the first time, because of all this legal shit between my mother and him, that maybe he had a reason not to believe this program was for real. So, I told him, OK, I'll send a copy of it."

Taking his father seriously for a minute allowed them to start speaking more over the phone. Dad took his time, gave somewhat less money than Walker (or Mom) wanted, but their relationship changed. The fights that had characterized previous communication began to ease.

It was not surprising that after this change with Dad, Walker's greater ease with his male friends became increasingly apparent.

*   *   *

Challenging kids to "speak the unspeakable" and not accept stereotypical views of parents helps them connect to themselves and others. Pushing kids to think ahead changes old behavior and possibilities. It lessens lying, along with the paranoid distance that comes with it. Challenging kids to empathize with their parents as three-dimensional human beings—how *they* might be experiencing the situation—turns the ruthless teen greed of a culturally induced divided self into deeper understanding.

Becoming Passionate about an Interest

Many years ago I worked as a camp counselor with a dozen 10- and 11-year-old boys. I was a college freshman, long before I had any training as a child professional. By pure chance, each boy had serious vulnerabilities. One was a bed wetter. Another had a terrible stutter. Another couldn't stop talking and was constantly sarcastic, to boot. One was almost legally blind and wore very thick glasses. One was effeminate. Another was a child who couldn't control his anger and regularly flew into tantrums.

Amazingly, within two months the kids moved beyond these problems that had for years significantly determined their sense of self. How? First, I tolerated no verbal abuse toward each other. Insults were absolutely forbidden. A few immediately lost privileges when they tested me. But I meant business. Along with this rule, I found the edge of relatedness each boy needed to feel a connection. I built little rituals around them—two-minute improv skits after lunch, an arm on a shoulder walking to dinner, writing cards home together, crazy mud-fights whenever it rained a lot, sitting by beds each night, or singing a lullaby, bad voice and all, until they dropped off to sleep.

As a climate of safety evolved, I began to recognize that each boy had hidden interests. *And, I figured that if they could be helped to develop these interests, they might end up feeling a little better about themselves.* For example, the boy who stuttered found it tough to mix it up with the other kids. However, he was very interested in the "audiovisual" department of camp. I set him up running movies and other technical matters that were essential to camp life. The boy who wet his bed happened to be an excellent athlete, in fact, a potential leader. But his bed-wetting made him feel damaged and babyish. I appointed him to be captain of our bunk team. The boy who was effeminate secretly loved baseball, but his lack of coordination sidelined him during sports, advertising the fact that he was not a "boy-boy." Every evening behind the bunk, we'd quietly throw the ball around for just a few minutes. The kid who was so sarcastic also happened to be a natural storyteller. I decided to encourage his aggressiveness in a more productive way: Tell kids scary bedtime stories at night.

Each boy dug into a talent or interest, and each became identified as being good at something. The truly amazing development was that as these stigmatized, wounded kids felt safe and worked on an interest, they actually got *a lot* better. By the end of the summer, the stutterer who had been to many speech therapists in the course of his young life stopped stuttering. The bed wetter, who had been plagued with this problem for years, stopped bed-wetting. The other boys would help strip his sheets in the morning; after a few weeks, the bed-wetting disappeared. The boy who had been flamboyant learned how to throw and catch the way a "boy" throws and catches. He was then targeted far less by campers from other cabins. The boy with the thick glasses joined forces with the stutterer to become our official audiovisual team. "Mr. Sarcasm" became a proficient storyteller. He was in such demand for his scary yarn-spinning talent, he had little time or interest in pushing people away.

I watched these kids transform. The director of the camp was stunned, as was I. Equally important, my own passion to enter the field had been ignited. Unfortunately, it took many years of *unlearning* some graduate school theories to get back to the kind of healing I unwittingly promoted that summer.

The Crushing of Passion

The kiddie culture has defined passion—to be enthusiastic about learning—to mean that you are not cool. TV, magazines, movies, music lyrics, and middle and high school cliques typically portray kids with passion as geeks; they are rarely in the cool crowd.

This observation is supported by longitudinal research. The Johnson Institute followed tens of thousands of kids and found that they tend to give up interests during the transition between elementary and middle school. It's very upsetting when parents watch a child who had once been a gung-ho artist, an avid piano player, a serious gymnast, a dedicated figure skater, or a committed student let that passion fall away at the dawn of adolescence. Not a week goes by that I don't meet a discouraged mother or father who describes to me an interest their child has dropped during this transition.

This phenomenon has become "culturally institutionalized." Passion requires a lot that is not part of second-family life—an ongoing relationship with an adult mentor, an ability to delay gratification, the necessity of prescheduling blocks of time, a willingness to stick with rigid rules, *and* an openness to a diverse group of kids—not necessarily those in one's inner circle of peers. So, parents watch helplessly (or become "fanatically obsessed") as their kids slip away from interests toward pop, TV, the Web, e-mails, chilling, teen movies, and getting the right stuff. This is one of many painful, but overlooked, losses that parents of teens must endure.

It is a challenge for us to ignite adolescent passion and go against institutionalized cool. To reconnect a teen with non-pop culture interests helps heal the divided self. It promotes the expression of the true self lying dormant within; it crowds out endless preoccupation with appearances and, as I first learned decades ago, sometimes even ingrained symptoms themselves. This is not easy to address. Most therapists do not focus on interests; we focus on problems.

Why Passion Matters

PASSION TEACHES KIDS THE PROCESS OF LEARNING

During my early years as a psychologist, I was influenced by progressive education that uses a child's personal interests to teach many of the skill-sets he or she needs. This approach is by now part of the curriculum in many schools around the country. For example, a child's love of baseball can teach reading (newspapers, magazines, books), writing (about a player or an aspect of the game), doing math problems (computing statistics, functions, even probability), and so on. Much can be taught by activating a passion, especially with teens in trouble, because they've been primarily organized around passive, consumer-oriented, second-family interests. I've watched a love of carburetors lead to friendships— other kids who liked cars; more first-family connections—fixing the automobiles of relatives around town; and a growing ability to be verbal—first about mechanical matters, then friends, then hidden feelings.

STRENGTH IN ONE AREA CARRIES OVER TO OTHER AREAS

Infancy researchers such as Dan Stern describe "cross modal" learning. When a child takes in information through one channel, say visually, learning can shift to another modality; in other words, she can be taught the same lesson auditorily. With adolescents in treatment, learning skills in one activity may spread into other arenas, and, of course, into growing self-esteem. The outcast, nasty teen who loves video games enough to pour over endless manuals begins designing Web-pages and school Websites. Occasionally she might even begin to read some schoolbooks, write lengthy e-mails, and, finally, a term paper.

DEVELOPING A PERSONAL INTEREST HELPS TEENS
GAIN PATIENCE

Becoming good at something is an antidote to cultural attention-deficit/disorder (ADD). Phrases such as, *"Obey your thirst!"* and *"Just do it!"* tell kids they should expect to get what they want *immediately.* High-speed Internet, Googling, surfing the Web, video game graphics, special effects, movies on demand, burning CDs, TiVo, and so on make it possible to switch from one fast-moving image to another without personal effort. All this creates the ability to self-regulate frustration and minimize nanoseconds of boredom. There is little to suggest to kids that even small steps lead to mastery, that frustration and dull moments must be tolerated before you get what you want.

Learning experts call this kind of boring work "skill acquisition," and life is about trying. *True-self desires almost always require effort, so much of treatment is challenging kids to move beyond pop culture habits, reconnect to their desires, and forge ahead through difficult periods.* As Adam (in the process of failing out of yet another school) said to me, "Everyone makes this all so complicated. The truth is I got used to the remote. I never got into the routine of doing work. It's as simple as that." Adolescents possess a natural predisposition to become "crazed" or "obsessive" or "mad" about something or other; they are not ones to do anything halfway. Our work with teens ought to counter the culture's pressure to divide them from their own true-self needs, and to instead worship the external façade and the appearance of things.

BECOMING GOOD AT AN INTEREST DEFINES A TEEN
IN THE SECOND FAMILY

When kids develop interests, their accomplishments define them in healthier ways. They become *known* for a particular skill by other kids, a minor celebrity of sorts. This identity is gradually integrated as part of the self. *The more kids are known for a specific passion, the less they act out* in response to what Michael Balint referred to as "the basic fault," an inner emptiness. For example, acting out had become a major way to fill Maya's inner void. After several months in treatment, Maya's outrageously provocative identity—neon hairstyle, Goth clothes, multiple piercings, and scathing words—were slowly crowded out by her growing visibility as a high school reporter and writer of scathingly realistic fiction. Adolescent angst and emptiness is sometimes filled when kids develop a genuine passion and become known for it.

Fostering Passion

REMEMBER TO ASK ABOUT INTERESTS

It bears repeating: At the very first meeting, ask about interests—no matter how serious the presenting problems are and even if a child is mandated into treatment. Also, get some rough idea of what his or her interests *used* to be. By the time many adolescents reach your office they have abandoned activities that were once enjoyable.

Although traditional training ignores this, a lot of nitty-gritty discussion with teens does not involve difficulties with parents. Nor do most professionals or teens talk only about the problems that originally got kids referred. As the relationship progresses, kids move from seemingly mindless pursuits—popularity, pop, gossip, celebrity—to friendship, love, school, and parents. Ask a teen what his current interests are and even mute clients become talkative.

Fifteen-year-old Hank was acting out in school as well as cutting almost all classes and, instead, hanging out in bars. He had been labeled by his teachers and counselors as subnormal in intelligence. Nonresponsive and impossible to engage, Hank was considered incapable of extended dialogue or insight. I, too, was on my way to failure until one day, mainly out of frustration, I asked Hank, "Hey, what are you really interested in? Forget the usual stuff. What do you like to do?" Following a long pause, Hank mumbled something about "cars." After a while of my pulling teeth, it turned out Hank absolutely loved everything to do with automobiles. This mute adolescent had endless knowledge of automobile life—models, engines, carburetors, specs, on and on. That one question led to many easy conversations—about cars. Through these discussions I learned who Hank's friends were, who he worked together with on cars, who he had trouble with in his life, and what his real difficulties were in school. From that point, we never had a meeting in which Hank didn't have something to say. Hank did not graduate high school. But he stayed out of deeper trouble and ultimately created a life that made sense to him.

By immediately inquiring about interests you set the groundwork for an experience that includes desire—not just difficulty and disappointment.

ENCOURAGE TEENS TO BRING THE WORLD INTO YOUR ROOM

Open up the walls of therapy to the artifacts of teen life—e-mails, video games, music, writing, photography, drawings and art—*and to their friends* (more on that later). Kids find it natural to bring in life and engage in a kind of adolescent show-and-tell. By sharing their artifacts, you set the stage for the development of an interest.

Ian was falling way behind in his schoolwork, and occasionally tearing apart his room in fits of rage—the latest event being a wild baseball bat confrontation with his mother. It turned out Ian was deeply engrossed in an online Internet strategy game about world domination, a game that involved a community of literally thousands of people. Ian played on revolving teams and got to "know" many of these kids in cyberspace. When he brought in this world, he spent much time explaining the complex strategies of the game, which fascinated me. One of the reasons Ian was having difficulty in school was because his online life was so engrossing, a second family of adults and kids with whom he played far into the evening. This siphoned off his energy and already-diminished motivation. Discussing this world and demonstrating it to me opened a window and led to Ian forming a cyberspace team in school. This was Ian's first move back into the academic arena. Over time his healthy need for mastery gradually shifted toward a growing interest in math—far away from the verbal skills he had such difficulty with.

Lizzie played songs every session on my boom box, bringing in her CDs so she could talk to me about how hip-hop music was different from gangsta, which was different from grunge, which was, *of course*, different from heavy metal. I let Lizzie teach me about music. Lizzie could make predictions about which group was going to make it and which wasn't. This was tremendously important to her, because Lizzie was seen as an absolute zero in school. Teaching me was a way to develop a sense of respect for herself—which led to becoming an intern at a small community college radio station. Over time, she developed into one of the few female DJs in her town and began to play music at school and private events.

Civilization: Items to Encourage Kids to Bring into the Room

- E-mail discussions
- Journals
- Favorite magazines
- CDs
- Video manuals
- Works in progress-hobbies, writing, projects
- Photos of friends, events, and trips
- Websites
- School magazines and newsletters
- *TV Guide*
- CD liner notes

MAKE PASSION AN ONGOING THEME OF THE WORK

When you ask a child what she likes you express an attitude, a way of connecting around passion that can slowly become a major treatment theme.

Juliet was 14 years old when I first met her. She was dealing with an affective/anxiety disorder. Despite being magnetic and sharp, she was a lightning rod for her small town's teenage turmoil. Fights, misunderstandings, and accusations constantly swirled around her. Even worse, Juliet felt secretly so empty and fixated on celebrity, appearances, and the pecking order of popularity that she flirted with self-cutting.

Juliet arrived with tapes of music to play on my stereo. It wasn't so much the music she enjoyed, however; the lyrics really got to her. From CD liners, she would read lyrics she found interesting or telling. Juliet started to collect some of her favorite songs in a journal; the journal slowly expanded to include e-mail conversations, especially passages from particular people she looked up to, phrases she found to be wise or cool. Interspersed with all this, she then began to keep a journal of her own thoughts and observations—the first written expression of her own inner self.

Juliet arrived for one session with printouts of a recent e-mail argument. It was clear to me at once how well she was able to express herself. Like many kids she perked up at my interest in the nitty-gritty details of her life. Slowly, as I reacted to the style as well as the content of her communication, writing became a natural theme of the work. Juliet realized that I genuinely enjoyed her ability to express teen angst in writing, and she brought more and more of it in. Almost every session, Juliet read parts of her journal to me. They revealed her shifting moods, in particular the many ups and downs with her friends. Sometimes, she'd enact these conversations, literally playing out parts of an entry or e-mail for me in the room.

Soon non-angst-filled letters to special friends appeared. Then writing reached across the divide—it became her way of talking to her father, leaving notes and writing e-mails to him about touchy teen subjects. Relationships with several teachers began to form around their appreciation of her work, as Juliet slowly developed the courage to show off her true self. Slowly, the theme in the room became the organizing theme of her life. Juliet realized that through writing she was able to calm herself down and gain perspective on what was happening. She'd write dramatic letters to friends that she had no intention of sending. Juliet had stumbled into an activity that was not only a passion, but helped soothe her moods. Writing was instrumental in allowing Juliet to handle her erratic emotions. She engaged in much less acting out and had fewer scathing fights with friends and family.

*　*　*

Logan loved music and took guitar lessons. He also hated school, was intensely self-conscious with peers, and had taken to smoking pot almost every day. Sometimes he'd bring in his guitar and play for me. We listened to his CDs on my boom box, and he taped music at home he wanted me to hear. Logan's interest in music developed into a theme—from discussions of the best bands—to talk about the possibility of playing "gigs" in his school. He formed a garage band with a group of boys and girls. As they practiced and practiced, Logan developed a *slightly* greater tolerance for studying. The group was good enough to put out a very cheap CD that the kids' families all chipped in to produce. Months turned into years, and Logan's interest evolved into a direction. Eventually he applied to a college conservatory for sound engineering. Logan had gone from being an alienated young adolescent to a young adult beginning to know who he was and what he loved in life.

*　*　*

Jon loved video games and, like many other unmotivated adolescents, practically memorized their elaborate manuals. He had been caught vandalizing buildings and arrested for graffiti writing. He was, not surprisingly, on the verge of failing out of school, having antagonized every teacher with his broken promises and almost every peer with his menacing distance. In this morass of dangerous behavior, my interest in his video manuals became an integral theme in our discussions. What began to emerge was Jon's ability to *think* like a computer. In time, he began to build and repair real computers. First, this was just for himself, then for a newly found group of friends. Jon became known for this talent by kids and eventually the teachers he so disliked in school. Serendipitously, the school was in a crunch—they needed a simple Website but had no money to underwrite it. Guess who? Jon volunteered to develop the site. The administration and his teachers were stunned, as was I. But we were no less shocked by the next development. Repairing broken machines was the tip of the iceberg—he didn't just fix electronics, he turned out to like helping others, and gradually became known as the "go-to" guy when one had an emotional issue. The theme of tending to technical needs slowly developed into a true-self desire to help others. There were many twists and turns on Jon's road, but he eventually became connected to his inner self and the world of people.

*   *   *

Collette was a 13-year-old seriously depressed girl even though she looked "perfect" to everyone else on the outside. Collette wouldn't act out with the other kids; she thought their weekend debauchery was stupid, and adults even stupider. Her nasty fights with peers drove her mother and father to despair. Collette considered herself to be an antihero and against anything that seemed tainted by self-interest. *The one activity Collette did relish, however, was arguing.* Take a position, and she immediately took the opposite one—a propensity not too appreciated by her peer group. I thought of Collette's arguing as her *interest*, and so our sessions took the form of constant debates. Here, in part, is how one sounded:

COLLETTE: Every adult I know is unhappy. My parents, all their friends. Probably even you.

THERAPIST: Why are we—they unhappy?

COLLETTE: They hate their work. They hate the institution of marriage. They hate everything.

THERAPIST: How can you be so sure of what they feel? You're saying you don't know one adult who's anything but unhappy?

COLLETTE: Well, just about no adults. No, I would say definitely not one. Anyway, what's your definition of unhappy?

THERAPIST: You brought it up, what's your definition?

COLLETTE: Well, an unhappy marriage.

THERAPIST: How are you defining an unhappy marriage?

COLLETTE: Not being happy all the time.

THERAPIST: So, you're telling me being happy means being happy all the time, every single moment. Then, I would have to say that, yes, you're right. Absolutely everyone I know, including me, and you for the rest of your life—everyone is unhappy now and is going to remain unhappy forever.

COLLETTE: No, don't be so dense. I don't think everyone is so unhappy every moment of every day.

THERAPIST: But you just said that. You said everyone is unhappy all the time.

COLLETTE: Well, my parents are mostly unhappy.

THERAPIST: OK, mostly is different. I know they fight a lot, but that doesn't mean everybody else, every adult you know, which you can't help becoming one day, is unhappy.

COLLETTE: Oh, I can help it all right. I can help becoming an adult. I just don't have to go with adult values, like working in school or, like, taking it seriously or getting involved with anything extra—it's futile.

THERAPIST: So you're saying everything is futile, everyone is unhappy. . . .

COLLETTE: I'm *not* saying everyone is unhappy!

THERAPIST: Well, let's say mostly everyone is unhappy most of the time, it's all futile—then it's no wonder you just lose yourself in reading fantasy fiction and don't get involved in school.

COLLETTE: How do you define reading?

Then we were off to the races again, lost in yet another argument.

Just about every session proceeded in this manner; I would either tear my hair out in frustration or sometimes enjoy the sport of it. One day, "just by accident," Collette dropped by the debating club at school. The head of the team told her, "Look, you can't really try out for this unless you get better grades." Collette came away grumbling; she and I argued about this "senseless" requirement next meeting. But she started to go to a few more classes, and got just enough Cs and Bs to be part of the team.

Needless to say, Collette was a terrific debater; this was her passion. Over two years, the debate club introduced her to a new world of like-minded, iconoclastic kids. Collette made the public school travel debate team. She started to go to matches in different countries, taking hundreds of pictures to document her journal, which led into another interest—photography. Collette's ability to debate was only second to her sardonic humor, appreciated by her peers. She was elected president of the debate team. Two years later, a boyfriend followed, someone she really loved, and one who became her first sexual partner.

As I described in Chapter 1, when kids get "better," they get "worse." The content of my meetings with Collette was now in the realm of high-risk behavior: sex, experimenting with drugs, nasty alliances, which kids were in danger, and which were OK. Collette's passion connected her to the darker side of the adolescent world, a development that often made me miss the safety of our endless debates.

*   *   *

Nia, a very anxious girl, and occasional self-cutter, was "the odd girl out" (in the words of Rachel Simmons) in school (*Odd Girl Out*, 2002). Over many years, she had developed an elaborate fantasy world derived from *The Legends of King Arthur*, the works of J. R. R. Tolkien and Phillip Pullman, and TV soaps. (Like Nia, boys have their own *Star Wars*, anime, Marvel Comics, etc., resources for their fantasy lives.) This was Nia's interest. In a sense, it was the reason she'd been brought to therapy. Although her parents didn't realize the depth of Nia's involvement in her fantasy world, they were concerned that she was fighting with other kids and didn't seem to have any friends.

Nia and I rarely talked about her presenting problems. Instead, all we really discussed were her fantasies. Nia kept two or three huge journals in which she wrote down the goings-on of her fantasy life, including pictures she'd drawn of the main characters. We'd spend the session discussing the attributes of these characters, which, of course, were attributes she felt she lacked in real life. She did have a couple of friends, boys who were also into elaborate comic-book fantasy worlds; occasionally Nia brought in their drawings, as well as the kids themselves to meet me.

As Nia explained her inner life to me, she turned into a master storyteller. This was what we built on—her ability to tell stories, to provide intricate details, and to spin a yarn. Somewhere along the way, Nia began to work with younger kids in after-school and summer programs. She signed on to be a mother's helper for difficult or shy kids. And, always, Nia would tell them stories. She was a hit.

I continued to see Nia from the time she was about 12 until she went to college. Less and less discussion was spent on her private fantasies, and more on the typical, but very worrisome aspects of teenage life. Nia became known in the world of peers and school as someone who was really good at describing ideas. Her growing confidence brought Nia out socially; she started to connect with friends and get invited to parties, and she turned into a wildly active kid. Once again, I now had to worry about a whole other set of problems—pot smoking, casual sex, weekend drinking, piercings, and intense panic about college—all the elements of normal adolescence that now made up her real world.

*   *   *

Passion is far from the only subject talked about in meetings. The rest of adolescent problems in living—ups and downs with friends, difficulties at home, trouble in school—are expressed along with or through passion. It becomes a theme. It becomes a concrete expression of inner self: who she is, how he is learning to define himself.

Watching secret passion and public self become integrated is extremely exciting. Becoming good at something heals the culturally induced divided self of adolescence. In fact, when a teen does not respond to challenges—opening up, becoming more empathic toward parents, or developing a passion beyond the pop culture, it is often a serious diagnostic sign. Contrary to negative hype about adolescents, it takes an awful lot of 21st-century culture to entirely divide teens. It takes a lot to squelch true-self needs—to be known to friends and even parents. It takes an awful lot to crush teen compassion and the drive to become really good at something they love.

It is a struggle to go against this powerful social current. And, during this struggle, adolescents, contrary to how we have been trained, need for us to give them no-nonsense advice.

5

DIRECTION

Advice as Essential to Helping Teens Change Behavior and Attitudes

Professor Dumbledore, Marge Simpson, Xzibit, Gandalf, *American Idol*'s Simon, Madonna, Limp Biskit—not exactly teens themselves, but kids pay attention.

T he story bears repeating: *Fifteen-year-old Mary says, "I went to the guidance counselor because these kids keep saying horrible things about me and threatening me. I wanted to know what I should do. So what does the guidance counselor say? She says, 'Tell me what you think you ought to do.' Do you believe that? Why the fuck does she think I asked her in the first place? What is it with you people anyway?"*

* * *

Mary is right. Advice is an essential part of engaging adolescents. It is glue in a relationship with kids. It creates a vital, mentoring exchange with an adult that helps a child feel held and guided toward better decisions in life. Yet traditional treatment and cutting-edge interventions with adolescents do not emphasize advice as integral. After speaking with thousands of mental health professionals, though, this supposed absence of advice is a sham. In fact, most of us offer a lot more commonsense opinion to kids off the record than we admit. Feeling as if we are doing something wrong by providing advice will certainly not increase our effectiveness with kids. Why are we so ambivalent about this basic reality of treatment?

WHY MARY IS RIGHT

The dilemma about ordinary, ongoing advice stems largely from the time-worn notion that a client ought to arrive at his own insights. He hasn't come to treatment to be told what to do. It is enough to vent or experience cathartic insight or develop an empathic relationship or rewrite the narrative of his life. More contemporary interventions are powerful approaches, indeed, but none *emphasize* direct, commonsense guidance about the ordinary details of daily living. Yet, in relationships that must help with the astonishing array of "normal" high-risk teen living, nothing less than full advice—from one of the few adults in a teen's life—will narrow the gap between second-family kids and the professionals who treat them.

WAIT A MINUTE. . . . DO TEENS EVEN WANT ADVICE?

A second aspect of the clinical dilemma is that adolescents are not known to graciously *accept* adult guidance. Professionals who deal with teens—therapists, school psychologists, counselors, clergy, and caseworkers—understandably worry that as soon as one tells an adolescent how to address a particular issue, she is likely to do the exact opposite. Adolescents, we have been taught, are resistant to any direct input from adults. Our own personal experiences as kids who may have fiercely dismissed the guidance of elders leaves its mark on our clinical attitudes: "Hey, I didn't listen to a word my parents said, either!"

ADVICE MAY BE RISKY BUSINESS

Even if we wish to offer opinions, professionals are increasingly *scared* to give advice. We may know that the high school boy sitting across from us should hear "You and your girlfriend need to get tested for HIV." But, living in a litigious society, some of the stands we take with young clients put us in vulnerable positions. In serious situations, it is likely that a parent will demand explanations and accountability—"Why wasn't I told this was going on with my child?"—and, perhaps, create a legal consequence: "Aren't you condoning his sexual behavior by sending him to an agency that does family planning and offers abortions? . . . The next person you will hear from is our attorney!"

The Case for Advice

Most clinical theories about working with kids were formulated during post-Victorian times. Treatment models evolved out of a fundamental notion that children were typically raised by an overcontrolling culture and parents. The therapist's task, then, was to pry teens loose from their rigid families. A hemmed-in child might well arrive at one's door needing to differentiate from an oppressive establishment. Tightly squeezed by nuclear families, monitored by extended kinship networks, lectured to by organized religion, contained by formalistic rituals and neighborhood schools, and watched by Main Street shopkeepers, it made sense that a child professional *not* be another individual in a child's life telling him what to do. The clinical theory on therapeutic advice fit the times—then. It doesn't—now. Or maybe ever again.

The context has changed so radically that adult advice as an integral part of dealing with teens may be a slam dunk. Chances are today's adolescent is *not* oppressed by parents, or, in fact, by any grown-ups. Kids are *not* smothered by an overarching, adult establishment. On the contrary, today's parents are often very much caught up in their own worlds—preoccupied, driven, ever multitasking. Kids today register this lack of adult direction. Mary's outrage expresses what many teens feel when they finally cross the great divide between the child and adult world. We adults don't always *get* that regardless of their defiant or jaded presentation, teens need to be guided, a void needs to be filled.

Twenty-first-century kids are not usually in the presence of civilian adults, besides teachers, except in the form of professional child wranglers—those who lead after-school or sports or camp experiences. These adults are much like office temps. They change from year to year, semester to semester, program to program, teaching module to teaching module. Wonderful though they may be, such grown-ups do not create an ongoing relationship from which concrete opinions are regularly sought out.

ACCEPTING ADVICE AS AN INDICATOR OF PATHOLOGY OR PROGRESS

The absence of adult guidance shows. When I review hundreds of cases, a pattern emerges: *The less open to adult advice, the greater the pathology of a teen or his family.* Lost kids have had few experiences with adults who are able and willing to guide, who have useful ideas to share. Many of the kids we see believe the primary source of advice is the second family—the peer group or pop culture.

Child professionals must address the cultural, almost institutionalized absence of guiding adults. Kids need a counselor who is not afraid to offer suggestions, who actually has something to say and who knows how to say things in such a way that even teens will hear. Advice is a *"bridge"* between parent and child, between what a child feels and the decisions she must make. Absent advice, the helping relationship is empty, a recapitulation of negligence in our culture.

Now, are modern teens *so* different that they immediately thank you for your opinion? Of course not. But, as the relationship evolves, even the most pathological or obstinate teens become less resistant to advice. Gradually, they *seek* out your wisdom. Over time, they become able to think *between* sessions about your views. This shift is an indicator of traction, a signal that the change process is under way.

The question, again, is not *whether* to give advice to teens, but *how*, in a pop and professional culture that says we should not. Make no mistake—I mean to foster public dialogue about this (let's face it, even the most orthodox analysts secretly offer guidance to clients all the time), so that advice is not cloaked in professional shame or is something to be hidden in peer supervision groups or from one's supervisor. Advice needs to be "out-ed."

This chapter offers suggestions about how to enrich the teen–adult connection and further kids' lives by offering advice within the complicated context of a helping relationship.

Learning Style Counts

There is a basic similarity between the learning that happens in treatment and a child's "learning style" in school. It is ultimately the responsibility of adult professionals to grasp a child's unique way of processing information. Mel Levine—author of *A Mind at a Time* (2002)—has influenced schools throughout the country. I've been a student and proponent of the "unique-minds" approach and have done hundreds of workshops in special needs schools over the past two decades. The message is simple: Instead of fitting children into wholesale educational models, we must fit what we are doing to match specific learning needs. A unique-minds approach is deeply relevant to all kinds of helping relationships.

Unfortunately, many therapists still think in developmental, post-Piagetian terms: Different developmental eras mean different processing. A unique minds approach shapes input to a child's emotional/cognitive learning style, increasing the chance that advice actually gets through. This matching often has more explanatory power than developmental, diagnostic, or clinical concepts. Following are some examples:

Twelve-year-old Ryan, extremely intelligent, had been having terrible difficulty with a boy in his class. Jeremy constantly picked on him until Ryan would publicly lash out. Many times I explained to Ryan why it was not wise to approach Jeremy and ask him a silly question, for example, "Hey dude, what time is it?" or even a sensible question like "What did the teacher say about our reading assignment?" Smart as a whip, Ryan simply couldn't understand how his behavior was being received by Jeremy—how it set him up for impulsive explosions and further abuse. His "resistance" to advice reflected a lack of social empathy; Ryan, smart about mechanical details and scientific facts (he had a history of developmental delays), could not get how his actions felt to Jeremy.

Ryan would respond to my advice concretely: "It was OK to ask him. I just wanted to find out about our homework." My attempts to explain rarely got through. In fact, given his language-processing issues, Ryan was hearing almost the *opposite* of what I meant: "Yes, sometimes it's OK to approach Jeremy" or "Approach him with a smile on your face" or "Phrase the question in a way that's friendlier."

Ryan has trouble reading visual cues, such as how close or distant to stand from people. He also has difficulty hearing the intent of what is said by anyone, including me. (What makes us think kids' learning would be different in the consulting room than it is in the classroom?) In the course of counseling 100 Ryans, I've come to ask clients with nonverbal learning issues to repeat exactly what I said: "What did I just tell you? What did you just hear me say?" The more I did this with Ryan, the more I moved onto his learning channel. Slowly, my advice helped him become significantly more adept at schoolyard politics. The questions stopped; he ignored Jeremy, especially when Jeremy was with his friends—and Ryan began to find his own group to hang out with.

J.B., on the other hand, loved to argue. Not only because he was an obstreperous 15-year-old, but because arguing *was the way J.B. learned*. When I first began to work with him, I didn't understand his learning process and how it needed to shape my advice. Unbeknownst to his parents, J.B. had started to drink, going to one of those teen-frequented restaurants that didn't "card"—there are some in every city. J.B. could easily down 8–10 shots of hard liquor a night. Sensitive discussions about why this might be dangerous—it could be difficult for him to cross the street safely or he could well be leaving himself open to being mugged—weren't getting through. This was not just because of normal teen defiance or omnipotence, but because it wasn't part of a high-voltage debate. For example, to my cautionary advice about binge drinking he would say, "I figured out the exact number of drinks I can have without getting drunk. . . . I'm drinking slowly over four or five hours, I'm pacing myself. . . . Everyone knows they water down the drinks in that place anyway; they like to take advantage of kids," and so on.

Becoming less inhibited about arguing with J.B. fit his specific style of learning and opened the door to his more reasonable side. Therefore, I came up with endlessly different rebuttals of my own. Many of our debates involved getting J.B. to recognize all the minor accidents that "seemed" to happen after he'd been drinking. For example, he'd sometimes stumble or trip over himself. He became more awkward with the girls he was trying to impress. The days following a drinking session, he would not only have a hangover, but would worry and obsess more than he normally did. (This is a common reaction in chronically anxious kids.) My experience of our meetings at that time was of constant debate. However, J.B. would often return to our next session and remark, "You know, some of what you said actually made sense. I *was* more nervous for days." Invariably, it was just when I thought he wasn't listening at all that an opinion of mine got through to him.

I began to understand that J.B's arguing was a way of testing my engagement as well as the logic of my remarks. Obstinacy was a means by which he could become clearer about his own thoughts—a major reason his parents and teachers had always thought J.B. was impervious to their input. From our intense exchanges, he began to think that maybe it would be worthwhile to experiment with drinking less, find a comfort zone, and see how that felt. J.B. had slowly absorbed these advice-laden debates. This was the beginning of change. Looking back I see even more clearly that J.B. simply could not learn from an empathic adult. It was no surprise that his mom needed to alter her Woodstock generation, pseudotherapeutic, Earth Mother approach.

Another example of how cognitive style and developmental/ dynamic issues must be respected when offering advice follows:

Marlena was an attractive, street-smart, 14-going-on-40-year-old kid. For a variety of reasons, the most subtle being her learning style, Marlena craved gentle but "crystal clear" advice. Her familial configuration would immediately jump out as an explanation for this. After mother and father divorced, Marlena lived in two different households, with revolving sets of adults in her life. Marlena's parents, children of the '70s, were conflicted about what was good for their daughter. Shouldn't she be a hip kid, too? Is a little drinking such a bad idea? Life is filled with temptations and everyone has to try things out and "find their own path." What should they say to Marlena about smoking dope? What about sex? Isn't sexuality a part of life to enjoy? Mom and Dad had difficulty providing clear messages because of their own ambivalence, and because they equated strong adult opinion with old-fashioned rigidity.

Unfortunately, for Marlena, her learning issue centered on processing verbal and written input. Taking tests, she often misinterpreted ambiguous instructions; verbal questions that could be construed in different ways drove her crazy. Marlena needed clarity in order to hear. The worst kind of advice from me, then, would have been something fuzzy, even slightly ambiguous: "Well, it could make you feel better about yourself on one level or maybe worse in the self-esteem department if you hook up with a boy you just met." Marlena needed to be approached without any extra phrases or any hints of ambiguity. Instead, I learned to say, "Think about this fact—everyone in school is going to know exactly what you did with that boy. You're going to feel bad afterward, because of what you'll hear about yourself."

Marlena had a great mind; she was a clear, analytic thinker. But if advice was presented any more vaguely than this, she'd just tune me out like so much unwanted background noise.

Rice, 13, fought with her parents over just about everything— how many showers to take, where to put her shoes after entering the house, what to wear for school. Her belligerence was spreading into the classroom, where she was getting into struggles with teachers. My advice style with Rice had little to do with presentation of language, with debate, or with being crystal clear, as in the preceding examples. Rather, it involved figuring out "What's in it for Rice?" Rice's inability to infer, to look at the "big picture," was a cognitive vulnerability. She needed to see the immediate gratification that a certain behavior would bring. Not a very high-order approach, but it was Rice's way of learning and hearing adult input.

Collaborative dialogue that included advice sounded like this: "I think you ought to take a shower every other night. If you spend so much time arguing, is your mom in a better mood or a worse mood? Is she more willing to order those clothes that you loved in the catalog? Is she willing to go on eBay with you?" I didn't say this all at once, but many times in different ways. The frame was an "If . . . then" sequence that emphasized concrete consequences. "If you do this, then, what happens? If you don't argue, then are you more likely to get what *you* want—sooner or later?"

*   *   *

Ryan, J.B., Marlena, and Rice each had a unique learning style. The many learning needs we face mean that advice cannot be offered in a formulaic manner. You must find the channel that is open for each child. If not, your show will be cancelled.

More Details, Better Advice

The more details you have, the better you will be at getting through to an adolescent. As discussed earlier, details enliven the relationship. They also enhance our ability to be smart—not just another clueless adult.

Unfortunately, grown-ups, even professionals, steer clear of the details. The details of teen life are often too shocking, explicit, or raw to hear. Sometimes, just like parents who would rather not know, we figure we can't do much about it anyway, so we move quickly toward *affect or logic* and away from actions. The feelings or rationale involved may be more comfortable to discuss because real-life teen behavior and decisions are often mind-boggling. However, without details we are simply too dumb to be helpful.

Talking explicitly about graphic details is hard for many adults, even child professionals. We were young once, too—but in very different times.

Could you imagine talking to your parents about kids "hooking up" at a party? About blow jobs, group sex, genital piercing?

Could you imagine telling your parents that other kids pick on you because you're fat? Or that you're a "loser"?

Could you imagine talking to your parents about kids abusing pot, Ritalin, 'shrooms, Ecstasy?

Could you imagine talking to your parents about eating disorders, self-cutting, graffiti?

Could you imagine voicing concerns about your sexuality or coming out as "bi" or gay?

If you've answered "no" to most of these questions, you are obviously not a 21st-century adolescent. Thirty years ago, teenagers lacked the vocabulary, the openness, and, perhaps most important, the blessing of the culture at large to bring up such subjects with their parents. That is why many mothers and fathers today cannot imagine that *their* kids would ever be willing to talk to them.

They're wrong. In fact, graphic exchanges are precisely the kinds of conversations teenagers continuously have with one another. As much as they may reflexively run away or change the subject when we initially broach "hot" topics, most kids are not completely against talking about once-taboo matters. Some actually make impassioned speeches to their parents. They think their parents owe them these discussions! After all, they see numerous TV parents and kids having them every night of their lives. "The times they are a-changin.' " When it comes to teen–adult conversation, Dylan's prophecy has reached critical mass, ushering in a new paradigm of potential candor.

So, get the details. They allow you to enter into a dialogue with enough information to offer advice. Following are some illustrations:

Kathleen, 15, had been referred by her school counselor, who worried that she was seriously depressed. I followed the sequence of questioning with Kathleen that I described in Chapter 2. I asked about interests, her second family, and the specifics of her daily life: Whom did she talk to? Whom did she trust the most? When she was especially sad, whom would she tell and what would she say? The kids Kathleen trusted most were an established boy–girl couple she knew. As her depression became apparent, I advised Kathleen's mother to approach this teen couple for help. They turned out to be wonderful resources for all the professionals involved, helping to monitor her self-destructive mood (which passed), available to offer suggestions and validate my advice to Kathleen. This unusual "team" effort was possible by close attention to the details of Kathleen's life.

Luke, 16, like many teens I know, was trying to arrange an online date with a girl, Jess, that he'd never met. As I probed into the details of this—"Where is Jess from? What time do you go online? How much time do you spend talking? What do the two of you talk about? What are you hoping for out of this?"—it slowly started to become clear to Luke who this girl was in real life, not just in cyber-space. Jess came from an extremely abusive background, had been raped by family members numerous times, had had several abortions, and did not normally like people who were from suburbs in the Northeast. Most worrisome, Jess wanted to meet with Luke alone in a motel off an isolated road in another state.

The more Luke described the details, the more obvious it was becoming to both of us that this meeting "could" be dangerous. It was now possible for me to say in a credible way, "You know, this sounds dicey. . . . I don't think you should have this meeting without asking your father what he thinks about your plan. He has a lot of experience with computers and girls." After a few half-hearted objections to my idea, Luke finally did talk to his dad—who felt so "honored" to be trusted with such personal information, he handled the situation brilliantly.

HE SAID—SHE SAID

Getting into the details might seem more difficult if you're a male counselor dealing with a teenage girl or a female therapist dealing with a teenage boy. This is an "old-think" concern. Over recent decades cross-gender discussions have become much easier. Boys and girls begin hanging out with each other early, in day care or nursery school. The division between boy and girl groups in elementary school has also significantly lessened. During the early years, birthday parties are co-ed. Sleepovers for many kids include boy and girl participants. Preteen groups see movies together. Girls and boys play (some) sports together through longer stretches of childhood. By middle and high school, girls are fairly used to "chilling" with boys, and boys are more comfortable hanging out with and confiding to girls.

In addition to these real-life changes, boys and girls watch most of the same TV shows and movies, over which there is an enormous amount of cross-gender discussion. Everyday topics among second-family friends include issues that would shock many "old" folks—those over 25. As I've written for years, what *really* startles adults is how casually graphic schoolyard friendship can be:

BOY: Do you want to hook up?

GIRL: No, I'm not interested.

BOY: Yeah, well you can go lick my balls instead.

GIRL: Listen, where your balls should be, someone ought to put up a "vacancy" sign.

BOY: You sound like you're reading from some soft-core porno script, you skank-bitch.

GIRL: Listen, dickhead, the answer is still "No!"

Then they seamlessly move into discussing whether a homework assignment is due the next day or whether they'll be hooking up that weekend. (See Denizet-Lewis, *The New York Times*, May 30, 2004.)

Professionals have discovered that kids are now far more open to discussing the most intimate issues, even with opposite-sex interviewers. Sex researchers, especially those who work with preteens and adolescents, acknowledge that when questioning kids about sexual behavior their biggest mistake has been failing to allot enough time to the process. They are burdened by their own outdated views that modern kids will be reserved with adults. What they have discovered, to the contrary, is that today's teens are remarkably willing to open up on any subject. If kids are asked specific questions they will be relatively uninhibited about revealing graphic details of their lives. Today kids simply don't have deep inhibitions about discussing drugs, sex, and rock and roll.

I have had the same experience in the consulting room. If I am not afraid to ask very specific questions in the right ways, kids will tell me a lot more than they used to.

Sheila, 14, was trying to decide whether or not to continue hanging out with a local "hot" boy, a two-letter athlete. It was hard to turn him down; this boy was idolized by so many of her friends. With him, Sheila would gain entrée into the "circle of cool." But the price of fame was that she was expected to drink a lot of liquor and also go down on him in the process. Asking about the details of explicit experiences had not always been easy for me. Over time, though, I began to realize that much of the discomfort with Sheila and so many other kids *was my own projection*. They were far less squeamish than I was about discussing the nitty-gritty details.

The more Sheila and I got into specifics, the smarter I got. I learned that her "hot" boy would suddenly cool down. Right in the middle of making out, he'd leave the room to play videogames for a while. I learned that Sheila had to take her clothes off, but he refused to remove anything. He made sure all the other kids knew what had gone on within an hour of hooking up with Sheila. After a while, we both realized how empty Sheila felt during the experience. All this allowed me to offer better advice. "I know it's tempting, but I don't think you should be with him. Yeah, at first people are impressed. But it makes you feel horrible afterwards. You make *him* seem important—not you!" Paraphrasing her words: "The more you do for him, the bigger a dickhead he becomes." From that, we were able to talk specifically about how she might handle post-football game invitation: If Sheila drank "only" one or two drinks she'd be better able to gauge her feelings. If she'd stay with a particular friend who hated this guy, the friend would be able to strengthen Sheila's resolve.

After detailed discussion and my advice, we easily moved into the underlying content, what we usually think of as treatment. "What is your need for power about? Who are you really trying to impress? Do you ever feel like you stand out at home?" and so on.

Without concrete details and advice based on them, the relationship would have been hollow. Knowing the specifics allowed me to be informed and more real. Had I simply said, "Stop doing that," with no idea of exactly what happened in those moments, my advice would have had little impact. On the other hand, had I exclusively focused on Sheila's feelings or logic, our exchange would have been flat. If we had not struggled over the details, possible strategies, and specific interactions our exchange would have had little traction.

Giving Advice without Being Controlling

Another reason therapists (and many parents) are hesitant to give advice is that it smacks of controlling another person's behavior. It's a perfect match—adolescents do not want to be controlled and we do not want to be controlling. So, we rarely feel comfortable giving unambivalent "I mean it" advice.

However, it is possible to present your opinion in such a way that it will neither *be* nor *feel* controlling to a teenager. Rather, it will be heard as a suggestion from an informed, caring person with a great deal of life experience. Good advice to adolescents should follow these steps:

  1. *"Here's what I think . . . "*

Say exactly what you think. The second family holds back few punches; schoolyard talk is graphic; online chatter is down-and-dirty. In comparison, most therapeutic dialogue is like "Lite FM" to teens—ambient noise that doesn't even register. Be absolutely clear. That meant telling Sheila, "I don't think you should be 'star-fucking' this guy."

And to Luke: "I think this computer date sounds frighteningly dangerous."

To Rice: "Rice, fighting over whether or not to take a shower every night is what an eight-year-old does. You're a teenager, not a baby. And you're not going to get what you want from your mother if you keep up these battles."

Don't mince words. As my grandmother's senior citizens' support group was called: "Speak Your Mind!"

2. *"It's your choice."*

The most critical aspect of giving advice is to state your limitations. Say, *"I can't control you. I won't be there, I can't make you do or decide anything. Nobody can, including your parents, and certainly not me. So, despite what I'm telling you now, it's going to be your choice."*

Recognizing *our* limits (we always focus on limits for kids), makes adolescents hear advice in a different way. They understand the truth of what you are admitting and appreciate that you can be realistic. Compare this to "You *can't* smoke at the concert," versus *"I know I can't stop you,* but I don't think you should smoke at the concert."

3. *"This is what will happen if . . . "*

Stating consequences that may follow a teen's decision is critical to good advice. Adolescents, just like all kids, feel safer when they know there's a concrete parameter they can't push past. But how do you—not being your client's parent—impose real-life consequences? You can't! (This is part of your job when working with parents, covered in Chapter 8.) The consequences you *can* provide, though, are a no-holds-barred description of what your client's behavior will create in her daily life.

I use my experience as one who has lived life and read the research. I use my expertise having listened to thousands of different stories from kids. These resources, which we all have, get clients to think the situation through to the end—"If you do this, here's what might happen."

Bryan, 13, was getting razzed around school by a few boys for being a "techie nerd." They tried to take small items from his rolling backpack. One of the boys snatched a package of pens that Bryan's mother had given him. When Bryan chased after the boy, the kids started to make fun of him, punching and putting him down for acting so desperate to get his geeky pens back.

I told Bryan the obvious: I could not be there to hold him back, so he was free to chase after them every time. But I also tried to draw a picture of the peer consequences. I asked Bryan to imagine what the boys might say if they saw another kid actually dive for a pen on the floor in school. What would *he* think about that boy? How would he look crawling on all fours after a rolling pen? A half hour into this, Bryan began to realize what I was suggesting: how absolutely silly he looked, and what an easy mark he made of himself. Several of these discussions, including advice on handling unfair behavior (Bryan was, of course, right about their bullying and stealing) increased his self-awareness and created different behavioral options in the process.

Sierra and Harris were two extremely anxious teens who, along with many adolescents I know, drank more than their bodies could absorb. Emphasizing my inability to control their behavior, I was also very clear how much I believed they suffered from their decisions. I helped them to remember—to think through—how they felt following a weekend of heavy drinking. After a number of failures even recalling my words, both recognized that for the next three or four days, they were much more ruminative than usual. Over time, Sierra and Harris began to see the consequences and that my advice had *slight* merit. For them, drinking was not going to simply be an escape or a way to have fun. The aftereffects lasted for days. One meeting Harris said to me: "I don't like it. But you're kind of, like, on my shoulder. When I have to decide whether to take that last shot of tequila, I think about what you've been saying, what might happen to me."

Sierra confessed: "I hate that I'm so anxious I can't just let loose and drink like everybody else. But I also can't forget what you've been saying." When Sierra and Harris eased up on their weekend escapades, we could begin discussing how they used liquor to lessen their self-consciousness, to flirt better, and to bond with other kids. Advice didn't stifle our relationship at all. It opened up our discussions.

The Ultimate Therapeutic Consequence

Finally, there is one consequence you can wield—loss of confidentiality.

> "Sheila, if you continue to put yourself at risk for STDs, we're going to have to figure out a way to tell your parents about this."

> "Luke, if you absolutely insist that you're going to make a date with this girl in a motel, one of us—you or me—is going to need to tell your parents. I can't stop you. But I can do something about this situation, so it gets to be talked about at home."

Deciding to break confidentiality is the last stop on the advice train, the ultimate therapeutic consequence. It is a complicated decision and will be covered in Chapter 7.

"Stop It! You Sound Just Like My Parents!"

The helping relationship, at some point, reenacts the troublesome "dance" between parent and child. As you know, the dance is a repetitive interaction in which everyone realizes where it is going—but cannot stop. To some degree, repeating the dance is unavoidable. Behaviors that go on in the family are almost always elicited in your relationship. Because adolescents are so dramatic, they provoke adults into many of the same reactions they provoke at home. Mostly this is good; reenactments are guidelines for what needs to be addressed in the work.

Unfortunately, *because of this phenomenon we often end up giving advice in the same ineffective ways parents do*. For example, Leon had a very difficult time with schoolwork, a problem that could not be chalked up to learning or attentional difficulties. Uncharacteristically, I would find myself spouting ridiculous, authoritarian pabulum: "Leon, if you don't study and work hard, you're not going to get a good job after school. You're not going to make it into a good college. You'll end up drifting into low-paying work you'll hate." Perhaps the words weren't exactly the same, but my harsh tone—empty warnings and vague threats about the future—was just what Leon was used to hearing from his mother.

J.B., the boy who loved to debate, explained that as the middle child, he felt ignored by his parents. One of his siblings was an attention-getter. J.B. said: "As soon as we get into a good argument, my parents are sidetracked by my older sister. I lose them in a second." And guess what? I was uncharacteristically distractible with J.B. Even as I offered advice, I found myself paying scant attention to his reactions—going over lists in my mind of other things I needed to do, checking the clock repeatedly, thinking about other kids in my practice. No wonder my words fell on deaf ears.

These experiences tend to be inevitable, especially in the tricky realm of offering advice to teens. But mindfulness—that you might be reenacting a parent–child dance—can help you offer advice in different ways than the ineffective dances at home.

For example, with J.B., after several frustrating meetings, I began to question the dance we were in. I finally realized that if I did not focus entirely and face him eye-to-eye, J.B. was going to feel just as invisible he did in his family. This was one teen who needed my undivided attention before he could even begin hearing me. Once this was identified, I could also help his parents become more focused advice givers in his complicated, high-risk world.

Remember Rice, who wouldn't shower? Initially I was extremely impatient with her. My condescending manner undermined any advice I offered. Again, this was a clue to the dance at home. She had an older sister who was quick on the uptake, gave their parents no difficulty with the "stupid" details of life, and who didn't need rewards for simple expectations. Dad was subtly contemptuous of Rice's difficulty with the little things. So, as soon as I sounded brusque or even mildly irritated, Rice tuned out. Just like her dad, I didn't get why showering was so difficult for her *and* why a concrete reward for her effort mattered so much. I didn't hear that having to dry her wet skin caused real physical discomfort (a common holdover from early sensory-integration issues). It soon became clear how my ill-tempered advice mirrored the judgmental dance at home.

When You Are Not Getting Through

When advice goes repeatedly unheard and I am pretty sure it is not a reenactment of an unaddressed family dynamic, I consider two possibilities:

First, an undiagnosed syndrome—such as an attentional issue, anxiety disorder, obsessive–compulsive disorder, masked depression (see my article in *The Family Networker*, 1990), adolescent-onset bipolar disorder, language-processing vulnerabilities—or the sequelae of early developmental disorders such as sensory defensiveness, Asperger and Tourette syndromes. Obviously, these require evaluation by a specialist in the area. The second possibility is a *family secret*—infidelity, impending bankruptcy, addiction, or abuse—which if left unaddressed, impacts kids in the ways I describe in the following examples.

Remember, despite their cool presentation, kids *want* adult advice. When a child is consistently unable to take in your words, and you've thoroughly considered your presentation, it is almost always a sign of an undiagnosed condition or a family secret.

For example, Billy secretly engaged in high-risk behaviors for years: driving at breakneck speeds down rural roads, gambling for huge stakes when money was extremely tight in the family, and borrowing cash from a slightly more comfortable cousin behind his mother's and father's back. After a year of meeting with Billy—during which time I unsuccessfully tried just about everything described in these pages—I learned that both his parents, and, in particular, his mother, had been engaged (during the entire counseling period, no less) in extramarital affairs. As I later discovered, the couple's closest friends had been advising them both to put a stop to these relationships. They took no one's advice, much like Billy ignored mine.

Katie was a midadolescent, and she and I talked at length about whether or not it was a good idea for her to casually engage in sex with boys who were nasty to her or with kids she barely knew. Invariably she'd argue with a boy and then hook up with him. Katie explained away the rough tone as typical flirting and banter. Given the raunchy nature of everyday schoolyard dialogue, I believed her. She'd casually hook up and find herself being mistreated in such a way that she and the boy would publicly do battle for days—and then hook up again. No amount of discussion, reflection, advice, or empathy made a dent. In time, I learned that there was a mirror-image dance going on at home. Her parents typically had sex right after a fight. During the times they were feeling friendlier, they were sexually uninterested in each other—a fact not lost on Katie. She'd observed this sequence hundreds of times—fights, then a closed bedroom door. When I understood and addressed their dance, Katie finally began to think about what I was suggesting. Though her behavior did not actually stop, her involvement with boys who weren't treating her well slowly began to lessen.

*   *   *

Contrary to stereotypes, when advice isn't getting through to a teen, it is almost always an indicator of unaddressed issues—*not teen defiance*. As I pointed out at the beginning of this chapter, hearing your advice is a sign of progress in the work, and is central to any successful relationship with adolescents. Do not be fooled by theoretical orientation or by initially unresponsive teens into thinking that a helping relationship with adolescents can actually happen without putting your opinions on the line.

Advice strengthens the connection, but not without intense parrying and a lot of lying, even to you, a dedicated child professional who only means the best.

6

THE GRAY ZONE

The Truth about Lying to Therapists and Other Child Professionals

> What do I want as a teenager? I want to do everything; I want to drive, to smoke, to party with no adults around, to keep my own hours. What do I want? I want to be a normal teenager. And, I'll say whatever it takes to be one.
>
> —*From interviews conducted with teens*

Most therapists are trained to conceptualize treatment as a place to unburden, a safe harbor. In the relationship, or "container" as D. W. Winnicott called it, a young client is able to be honest. If she is *not* honest with herself or authority figures, she is conflicted about it, that is, she feels guilty about lying. Psychodynamically oriented clinicians have been taught that conflict between superego and unacceptable impulses eventually creates symptoms or security operations in nonsociopathic individuals. Systemic family therapists hold a similar view—symptom-bearing kids are distressed enough about lying that they often need to be caught acting out in order to bring the family into therapy. This sequence is usually interpreted as a cry for help, both for the child and for the family. Cognitive therapists use the concept of "schemas" to understand lying or deviant behaviors. Twelve-step counselors view lying as denial, the illness taking over an individual's nonaddicted self. A child's lying, then, is thought by psychoanalysts, family therapists, school psychologists, 12-step counselors and even pop psychology writers to be accompanied by *some* discomfort. Lying, as resistance. Lying, as conflict. Lying, as denial. Nonconflictual lying, as sociopathy.

But, what if these assumptions no longer hold true? And, for many contemporary teens they do not. Learning difficult lessons as a therapist, I have come to understand that dealing with non-conflictual, chronic lying is an essential part of teen treatment. For millennium kids, lying means something very different than it did in post-Victorian United States.

Some years ago, the following example caught my attention. Two sisters were in separate treatment. I was seeing Lynette, about 12 at the time; Carla was 17. Young Lynette was dubbed the good sister, while Carla was the bad sister. They were considered by parents and teachers to be the archetypical "angel" and "devil." Carla had never done well academically and, in fact, was about to be placed into the slowest track of the grade. Everyone identified her as a problem child who was disrespectful to her parents and teachers, saying anything she felt to them. Lynette was the exact opposite. She was a honey, a *good* girl who got straight As, was class rep in her student council, and was inordinately respectful to adults. In family sessions the therapists conducted with their parents, both acted true to form: Lynette was cooperative and polite; Carla was impossibly rude and difficult.

One day someone in their suburban hometown mentioned that Lynette had been seen smoking with a group of kids. One thing led to another, and it turned out that all the apparent roles were exactly the opposite. Carla was deeply worried about Lynette and intent on getting her to change. Carla, a "lying good-for-nothing" as her parents reported, was so worried that she had developed a chronic headache disorder. The older daughter considered herself of a different generation than her sister, aghast at how Lynette could so glibly lie and get over on all the adults around.

In fact, despite appearances, Carla wasn't behaving much out of line, aside from being fresh around the house. Her trouble in school was real. But eventually it became clear that these difficulties stemmed from an undiagnosed reading disorder. It was Carla's kid sister, "good" Lynette, who had been sleeping around, had been smoking pot, and was nice to the world of adults but absolutely hell-bent on acting out in the world of kids. It was striking that none of the adults knew; parents and kids were, indeed, living lives in parallel universes.

Discovering the truth behind the appearances was a crushing blow, since I had not suspected any of this. At the time I thought I was witnessing an isolated incident. I had not yet worked with enough adolescents and families, nor had I started speaking to tens of thousands of parents and professionals across the country. In addition, I chalked up Lynette's coolly calculated deception to being part of adolescence—because, really, what's new about teenagers lying? We can all think back to times we didn't tell our parents what they wanted to know; we lied to them about where we were going and what we were doing and whom we were with. So, although probably few reading this book were pure as the driven snow, the *quality* of teen lying has dramatically changed. And these changes profoundly affect what helping professionals must deal with today. By now, I have seen and heard about countless Lynettes.

ACTING OUT AND LYING HAPPENS AT EARLIER AGES

An example I have written about before—one that gives me a chuckle, but also opened my eyes—is this: Several boys were regularly sneaking into the basement of a friend's home, in a sleepy suburban neighborhood. They gathered to watch porn on cable TV. The eye-opener, for me, was not what the kids were doing. How many young boys don't feel pulled towards porn? The eye-opener was the fact that most the kids in the neighborhood knew what was going on, but *not one of the parents did*. The boys were 9–10 years old.

I remember another teen, a girl who was rushed to the emergency room after drinking an entire six-pack of beer in one evening. She was a gymnast, a very small child, and obviously her body could not absorb such a significant amount of alcohol. It was shocking to all the adults involved that she had done this, but even more shocking was that this kind of drinking had been secretly going on for a long time. Again, the kids knew, but none of the adults did. The girl was 12 years old.

Acting out and the complex second family network to back up a lie begin at earlier ages. Just a while ago we would have considered this behavior not at all common until mid-adolescence or later high school. National researchers tell me that the biggest changes in high-risk behaviors are happening in middle schoolers. Whether it is substance use, sexual experimentation, or simply the effects of peer pressure, "normal" adolescence starts earlier than it did just 10 years ago.

LYING ISN'T CONFLICTUAL . . . IT'S ABOUT BEING NORMAL

We were taught that there was almost always internal conflict in a child or adolescent who lied. Kids invariably needed to be "found out." For example, Coleen, a high school senior, with just one more class to finish, blatantly plagiarized an entire term paper— easily spotted by her history teacher, who had until then not recognized that Coleen had lifted many portions of writing from others. This put graduation at total risk. The incident landed Coleen and her family in treatment. Her conflict about secretly cheating ended up helping the family deal with their impending transition.

What is different now is that the thousands of child professionals I speak with see less conflict in kids, less internal guilt about what they've done. The wonderful "catharsis scene" from old movies or stories—the sudden confession about something one feels horrible guilt about—doesn't happen all that often in reality. Carla, the "bad" sister I described earlier, *did* feel guilty about lying. But she seemed a generation older than her kid sister. "Good" Lynette, on the other hand, felt absolutely no guilt at all. Although I didn't realize it at the time, I would be working with hundreds of kids who were much more like 21st-century Lynette than Old World Carla. The girl who drank herself sick, the boys watching porn in the basement, and the sophomores at sex parties are not racked with guilt. For the most part, they are not trying to get caught. On the contrary, they try as best as they can to get away with what they are doing.

We ask, why? Very few of these children are sociopaths. I follow kids for years after treatment. Almost every adolescent I've known eventually made it through second family life. They grew up to be good adults and decent citizens. Modern teens are not morally bankrupt. They don't even feel as if they are making choices between good or bad, or that their behavior is morally questionable. *Lying is simply a means to a justified end: to protect one's options—in other words, the right to a "normal adolescence."* This is defined as the right to have fun, to feel comfortable, and to be free. This is greater than any sense of guilt, and, as kids say, it is no different than the adult "culture of me."

Internal conflict and candor are not something helping professionals can anticipate. You can't count on a child spilling the beans because he is torn between id and superego, between crime and punishment, between guilt and guilt-ridden pleasure. "What's wrong" as kids often tell me, "about a right?"

NO ONE (ADULT, THAT IS) WILL KNOW, ANYWAY

Kids today are not particularly fearful of being caught or punished. In interviews with teachers, counselors, camp directors, and middle school and high school principals, I have heard the same story: The current (well-intentioned) emphasis on teaching morality, empathy, and social skills has limited effectiveness without consequences. "We need to bring back the idea," they repeatedly say, "that there will be a punishment to a 'crime,' or kids just continue to casually lie and act out."

Over the last five years, in workshops around the country and in my parenting book on adolescence, *The Second Family* (2001), I have underscored the belief that kids need a *balance* between empathy and expectation in their lives. What is important for child professionals to realize is that without worry or consequences, adolescents will not likely feel genuine conflict about lying.

Actually, getting caught is not even on most teen's minds. Lost in urban and suburban sprawl, city-sized supermalls and the far reaches of cyberspace—who in the adult world *knows* what goes on behind the wall of silence?

THE WALL OF SILENCE

The cybernetic revolution has increased kids' expectation of freedom like no other force. The Internet, cell phones, text-messaging, wireless communication, beepers, and pagers are endless, invisible ways to instantly get in touch with each other behind an impermeable wall of silence. Never before have so many kids spent so much time in worlds entirely uncontrolled by their parents. Angie said about her 14-year-old daughter, "She is online every night with friends whom I've never met and never will meet. I have no idea what a large chunk of her life is like. *I feel like I don't know who she is.*" (This 21st century parental lament—"I don't know *who* my child is"—differs from the older "I don't *like* my child since he became a teenager"—and is far more worrisome, more disconnected.) The vast, unsupervised world of the Internet is transforming not only the way kids experience their lives, but the way parents experience their kids—or fail to experience them.

The second family's wall of silence is astonishing; it is exactly what kids from previous generations wished for. But they could not quite accomplish it in a bricks-and-mortar age—with local shopkeepers, extended kin, and neighbors hovering nearby.

A young teen was referred to me because he had traveled halfway across the country to visit a girlfriend. We might say, well, adolescents will go to great lengths for love and lust. What was amazing about this boy's flight, however, was that his parents didn't even know he was gone. He had four or five backup plans in place, so that friend "A" said he was spending the night at "B's" home, and then friend "C" beeped him when the boy's parents called, so he could call them back from wherever he was at the moment (the double-edged sword of cell phones). It was three days before his parents figured out that their son was nowhere remotely near the town they lived in. Though this at first seemed far-fetched to me, I heard a similar story several weeks later that was even more stunning—a teen made it to Thailand without a single adult suspecting, and with just about every kid around in the know.

Thirteen-year-old Tanya says to me in passing, "Don't mention that Nell has a boyfriend because her mother doesn't know." Nell's mother didn't know because she worked long hours. But, more significantly, Nell met the "boyfriend" online; Mom had never heard his voice, had not ever seen him in person. Nell and he communicated in dozens of ways that her mother and other adults had absolutely no awareness of. This, while Nell's entire second family knew almost every detail of the couple's complex interaction.

Like so much else in their lives, kids are able to "self-regulate," in this case, the distance between the second family and the world of adults. A 24/7 connection with each other makes it possible for teens to live life the way *we wish we could have*—a second family to feel intimacy with, to back each other up, and a world of anonymity to hide in.

I often don't know whether I feel envious or scared.

Lying in the Consulting Room

Put this all together and lying is as commonplace in the treatment room as it is in the living room. Of course, our clinical sensibilities practically guarantee it. I would rather be a compassionate listener than create an atmosphere in which my client senses that I am scrutinizing him or her. I would rather err on the side of being "easy" than risk being a stifling adult. This ethic made sense in a post-Victorian world, a culture that *was* repressive. Kids truly needed a safe space to open up. Since the culture has changed so dramatically, we face a different challenge: *to create a safe space that is not blindly accepting.* Think back to how often you have been stunned to discover the reality about a child or family. The "devil" and the "angel" situation described earlier, was far from being the only time I was duped.

Ethan, 15, was referred because of an increasing malaise, a seeming lack of passion about any interests whatsoever. This was not one of those dramatic cases I thought I'd spend a lot of time worrying about. A year later, though, I discovered how wrong I was. Ethan was smoking pot two or three times a day. Since eighth grade, he had also been the local dope dealer. None of the adults— his parents, his teachers, or me—had any awareness of this double life.

Sixteen-year-old Marina, a case on which I consulted, was se-cretly bulimic for almost two years. Her parents and therapist had absolutely no clue. This reality only came to light when one of Ma-rina's bunkmates at camp became so worried that she broke the wall of silence and finally told her 18-year-old counselor what was going on.

In a case I was supervising, Marilyn, 14, was depressed. She had been actively cutting herself, and since she refused to change clothes in front of her mother, the scars couldn't be seen at home. Her closest friends, however, were aware of what Marilyn was do-ing; one of them finally couldn't take it anymore and after lengthy deliberation told the school counselor, who called Marilyn's thera-pist—who had also been totally in the dark.

Living in "The Gray Zone"

Almost every clinician I've spoken with feels caught in a bind working with high-risk teens—a bind they can't quite articulate, but one that makes complete sense. *The helping situation itself creates a terrible conundrum. We make it difficult for kids to be truthful, even though that is exactly what the relationship is supposed to be about.*

When an adolescent comes to treatment, we spell out the "if you or anyone is in danger . . . " rules of confidentiality. Under-standably, we need to make clear what circumstances might break confidentiality. At the same time, it puts the entire situation into a Catch-22, especially with high-risk, modern kids. It is a dilemma we haven't yet figured out how to solve, or even discuss—one that practically ensures lying on a teen's part.

The key to unlocking this dilemma is recognizing that "normal" adoles-cent behavior is gradually becoming "high-risk" behavior. A therapist with whom I consulted was seeing a 15-year-old who occasionally missed sessions, who was not taking his antianxiety medication regularly, and who was smoking pot instead. This boy was in the "gray zone" of danger. The therapist said nothing to his parents be-cause missed sessions, failure to take non-life-critical medications, and a little dope smoking failed to meet what he considered imme-diate danger.

But is it? A lot of what preteens and adolescents do these days is, by definition, high risk. For example, when does a teen's drinking or smoking become dangerous enough to force you say something to a parent? When does sexual acting out count as a dangerous situation? At a certain age? When the client is not having intercourse, but is engaging in other sexual behavior? Is it when a teen is sexually active, but is ignoring safe-sex practices? What about finding out that a client is going to a house where there is no supervision and the kids will surely be drinking and hooking up? What about a keg party, with half the neighborhood's kids involved? It's "normal," all right, but you may be the only adult who knows about the plans. Are these legitimate triggers to break confidentiality?

Since only kids understand the extent of what is really going on in the second family, they are well aware of just how dicey their exploits are. They also know we live in a litigious society. Some sense that confidentiality may be trumped by our concerns—legal suits, complex HIPAA requirements, managed care reviews, and so on.

DON'T ASK—DON'T TELL

For all these reasons, therapy—the place for potential honesty—is unintentionally structured to create a *"don't ask, don't tell"* paradox. Lying is not going to disappear in the presence of a benevolent professional who, for complex reasons, may not want to know that much more than the adults at home. Whether kids get all this or not, professionals certainly do. As a high school counselor admitted, speaking for many, "Sometimes, I'd rather not know. I may have to report; the situation will become burdensome on my time and maybe more dangerous for the very child I'm trying to protect."

How to Lessen Lying

What is the solution? *Taking the gray zone seriously short-circuits a self-perpetuating tilt toward lying*: The more kids omit or fabricate, the further they slip into the hidden world of the second family. The longer this goes on, the more high-risk behaviors are considered ordinary behavior. "Coming clean" with an adult may eventually mean talking about immediate danger, indeed, triggering a break in confidentiality and a precipitous loss of freedom. So, lying continues.

Paradoxically, the lower your threshold for concern—the earlier you openly struggle with your patient about gray-zone behaviors—the greater the traction before real danger threatens confidentiality.

What follows is a discussion about seeing the gray zone more clearly, even with glib teens, who are used to running circles around adults.

FORGET YOUR GOOD INTENTIONS

You represent the child's parents and the law. Despite those credentials proudly displayed on the wall of your office, you are an adult, who may be a threat to freedom. No matter how compassionate, you are a grown-up who is ultimately a threat to a teen's autonomy. *You must expect, then, that conscious lying will occur, in almost every session.* Your mind-set can no longer be that of a totally accepting person. Gullibility does not create connection with a second-family teen who is orbiting further and further from the universe of adults. Kids view ignorance with disdain—it increases disconnection.

Instead, you must be skeptical, difficult to fool, *and* compassionate.

I finally understood this "non-Rogerian" reality while meeting with a group of 14-year-olds, friends of a boy I was seeing in treatment. The kids began to discuss parents. It seemed that among these teens, one parent, and only one, was experienced as a substantial force. When I asked what made this father so different, they replied, "Because he knows that we're lying, he sees through us. It's sort of spooky that he can tell when we're being straight. None of the other parents get it. And they don't really want to."

Kids must come to see us as like that boy's parent. Not another clueless adult, but one who understands (without harsh

judgment), that good kids lie in treatment. *All* the time. To *all* helping professionals. This change of mind-set creates a very different
atmosphere, and it creates the potential for real connection. You
become one of the few adults in an adolescent's world who actually
sees past the façade and can talk about real things in their lives.

A final point about changing your mind-set: Try not to exces-
sively criticize yourself for failing to spot teen lies. In my own experience, these discoveries come out of left field, almost completely unanticipated. When you look back you realize that the
behavior was the last thing you would have predicted, and, in most
cases, the revelation was not just a mild surprise, it was an "Oh my
God!" shock. There are so many new worlds that kids are into, you
can't always imagine them ahead of time.

MAKE YOUR SKEPTICISM CLEAR AT THE BEGINNING OF THE PROCESS

By the end of the first meeting, I want to have gotten across the
idea that I am not totally gullible. I am not going to be a "Yes, yes, I
understand" therapist, accepting at face value just about everything that's said.

The way I bring this home is to "prescribe" the symptom of lying, a technique made popular by family therapists decades ago.
Remember the question I ask at the very end of the first interview:
*"On a scale of 1 to 10, how much of your life have you been honest about
with me? You don't have to share anything about what you've left out. I
know you'll have certain secrets. But, I also know you haven't told me everything. So, on a scale of 1 to 10, I want you to rate what you've said here
today."*

When adolescents hear this, they smile. Many kids will, for the
first time, look me straight in the eye. And they will give a fairly
honest answer.

Few teens have been offended by my friendly skepticism.
Rather, if kids want to fool me, which, of course, they can, at least
I'm not foolishly secure. Sixteen-year-old Jena responded to my
skeptical question with a long silence. Then we had the following
exchange:

Reality Check

Here are some other remarks I might make, depending on how truthful the session seems:

+ "I can guess from my experience that there are important things you've left out today. Just how important are they?"
+ "I don't believe that no one in your group has ever tried . . . "
+ "It's pretty unusual for teens to have absolutely no experience with . . . "
+ "In my gut, I feel . . . "
+ "If your friends were here, what would they say?"

JENA: I'm not going to answer that right now. (*Another silence.*) Do you see other kids my age?

ME: Yes.

JENA: Boys or girls?

ME: Both.

JENA: Wouldn't you rather *not* know what's going on?

ME: You're right, that's very smart of you. Sometimes I would rather not hear, but despite my worries, I'll take the chance.

JENA: (*after another pause*) Well, what about my parents knowing? . . . There's a lot I haven't told you.

ME: Take your time. . . . I didn't expect you to. And just tell me what you want kept confidential. We'll figure out together what's truly dangerous as it comes up. . . .

This teen-savvy exchange, taking place in the first moments of our relationship, had an impact. Jena heard several messages: (1) I was not entirely gullible; (2) she could talk about dicey behavior without my unilaterally breaking confidentiality; (3) she and I would grapple with issues of danger and confidentiality as we went along. *Confidentiality was not black or white; it was an ongoing, flexible parameter.*

Jena gradually revealed that since spring of eighth grade, she had been sexually active with both boys and girls (though still technically a virgin), had experimented with most recreational drugs, and had managed to secretly pull it all off because she was a straight-A student. With each revelation, we discussed whether and how her parents should know. This self-regulating aspect of the relationship "held" Jena. She was with a compassionate, but not entirely clueless adult.

PAY ATTENTION TO SMALL SIGNALS, NOT RED FLAGS

Part of working with teens is to *proactively* search for the truth. It will not be revealed by passively providing a safe container. Searching requires skepticism, especially regarding gray-zone behaviors, about which tiny details are always present.

The earlier you grapple with the gray zone, the less chance the behavior will turn into confidentiality-breaking danger. For example, an event explodes in the middle of treatment: A boy is caught driving with six friends at a speed of over 100 mph while intoxicated. A girl has life-endangering bulimia. Another has been mixing binge drinking and Ecstasy. Almost always, when you look back, there were tiny details you didn't pay attention to. Just like parents at home—now you see it; now you don't! How do you keep your eyes open when therapy is constructed in such a way that you cannot help having empathic failures, when you can't understand what is going on in exactly those areas that are causing your client the most trouble? As interpersonal writers point out, it is almost impossible *not* to miss just those issues that are especially problematic for our clients.

But teens are still teens. Secretive though they may want to be, a lot spills out. They are much more dramatic than most adults. If we keep our eyes open, kids leave a trail of debris. Despite their desire to cover things over, kids are not always great at attending to the flotsam and jetsam, the details of time and the intertwining stories of their overscheduled lives.

Here are some early warning signals that trouble is brewing beneath the surface. It is time to pay closer attention, so you can openly struggle in the gray zone, way before the confidentiality of treatment is threatened.

SOMETHING DOES NOT QUITE ADD UP

Sixteen-year-old Barry was always anxious about tests, for good reason, since he hated reading anything but video game manuals. At one point a major paper was looming, and yet Barry suddenly didn't seem quite as concerned, certainly not in the way he always had been. I remember a fleeting thought—"This is odd!" and, ironically, "Is he getting better because of our work?" I didn't pay much attention to this nanosecond of wisdom. It turned out that Barry was "borrowing" money from other kids to buy term papers. Of course he wasn't nervous. But my observation didn't register vividly enough before he created serious trouble in his life. He was suspended from yet another school for the behavior. He ended up in a Western wilderness program for acting-out kids—not bad for Barry, who needed a very tight watch over him. But what if someone had noticed earlier?

Adrienne, 14 years old, mentioned she was inviting a few friends over for a party. Her parents would be there, she said, engaged in household tasks, like doing laundry in the basement—which for a brief moment made no sense at all. Laundry, on a Saturday night? I asked how she was planning to control the party while her parents were otherwise engaged. Adrienne explained that a bunch of her friends had promised they would take care of crashers—it was to be a small gathering. This, too, didn't make sense, knowing how quickly word spreads in the second family. In fact, she had been secretly planning a blowout, expecting over 100 kids. The fact that her unsuspecting father was engaged in caretaking his brother's imminent death added a twist of ruthless, teen self-absorption into this everyday drama. To me, Adrienne's story didn't add up; a full discussion between us ahead of time significantly toned down the scope, the secrecy (she eventually spoke to her mom about it), and the danger of her plans. We were then able to discuss the impact of her uncle's chronic illness on family life.

Another high school girl, Cassie, talked to me about a trip to Myrtle Beach during spring break (a time-honored ritual once reserved just for college students), to visit her grandparents. She'd be going with her best friends. Her friend's mom and dad would be there too, so they'd be supervising the three girls. That didn't sound right to me. I knew a little about the families and I believed her friends' parents would not want to spend that much time cramped in a small hotel room with their kids. In fact, there were no parents to be found at all—the girl's grandparents were ostensibly in charge. These two elderly individuals had absolutely no idea about the 50-kids-at-a-time, toga, hose-drinking, orgy-like parties their granddaughter was planning. All of which would have destroyed the relationship between Cassie's mother and the equally unsuspecting parents of her friends. Our discussion of the details led to different vacation arrangements, which was fortunate—several kids in her grade landed in a local emergency room with alcohol poisoning.

When you pick up even the tiniest signals, you need to trust your reaction and to say in so many words: "You know something? What you're telling me just doesn't make sense." Direct observations on the issue of truthfulness are what make kids take notice. They feel they are in a room with a straightforward adult who is not going to accept a lack of truth, even if the rest of the adult world is. More important, gray-zone issues can be discussed, sometimes preventing them from moving over into the red zone.

THERE ARE TOO MANY REASSURANCES THAT EVERYTHING IS GOING TO BE OK

Seventeen-year-old Simon reassured me and his parents 50 times over that prom night was all set, offering elaborate details about many checks and balances throughout the event—designated drivers had already been chosen, specifically, kids who had never received a moving violation (a nice touch); one friend's parents were very strict; and they'd be calling in every hour. The number of his reassurances was inversely related to the fact that, in reality, there would be no supervision, no adults were remotely involved, and absolutely no adults knew the kids were planning to sleep on a far-away beach the next day. This was an instance where I had to break confidentiality indirectly by helping Simon's parents to "open their eyes" (see Chapter 8).

TO LESSEN LYING, BRING THE POP CULTURE INTO THE RELATIONSHIP

Another way to find out what is going on behind the façade is through the pop culture. Pop culture interests reflect kids' hidden concerns, what they are really thinking about, and what they're doing just out of sight. Pop culture, as an ongoing relationship theme, is a metaphorical way for kids to tell you secrets without actually having to say them out loud.

Zoe kept bringing in CDs of groups who sang about anarchy and nihilism. After several weeks this led into a halting discussion about her secret participation in a counterculture game called "Killer." Killer involves teams of high school kids who "attack, capture, or kill" each other. The game goes on 24/7. Though no real weapons are used (paintball guns are the weapons of choice), the game is outlawed by many schools, because the scheming, plotting, shifting alliances, and midnight captures obviously consume kids from morning till night. Without her songs as an easy introduction, I'm not sure Zoe would have ever discussed this taboo topic.

Video game paraphernalia offer another view behind the façade of the second family. Kids bring their manuals to our sessions. It is amazing that boys who will not read a single textbook haul in manuals 300 pages thick, filled with thousands of bits of arcane information they've completely memorized. The plot lines of these games tell me what kids are feeling, thinking about, and actually doing. My client, Carson, was an "outcast," a nerdy but rageful kid who felt chronically dissed by the jocks. Through a Web video game, he was developing elaborate ideas about how to get back at his tormentors. (It is astonishing, the number of kids online every day, making connections with other kids they've never met.) Until we began discussing the game in detail, Carson's cyberspace plots felt all too real. Talking about his video involvement allowed Carson's revenge to remain at the fantasy level. Slowly he joined the real world, becoming less estranged from kids in his classes. This is when *real* trouble began—staying out late and not coming home, active sexuality, bringing friends over to smoke pot in his empty house. Remember the myths in Chapter 1: As teens approach "normal," they are increasingly involved in second-family dangers.

Another source of information—outgoing phone messages, especially those of early to mid-adolescents, often contains telling descriptions of life outside the view of adults. In a case I supervised, the therapist reported in passing that her adolescent client labeled himself "Buddha" on his voice mail. This boy (as we found out later), was an accomplished dope dealer. Buddha is a not-so-secret code word for pot. The kids knew; the adults did not. "Cute" thought his parents: "He has an interest in Zen and Eastern religion." Meanwhile, he drifted further into the second family and behind a wall of lies. One day, a kid happened to mention this term to me, I finally realized its meaning and passed it on to the therapist. Another example: the seemingly meek and mild-mannered girlfriend of a boy whose family I'd known in my neighborhood since grade school had recorded his outgoing phone message: "Who the fuck are you—and what do you want with Adam—please feel free to leave a message." Jane was not as light-hearted or easygoing as her adult persona suggested, but a possessive, angry, and very persuasive 15-year-old. From these discoveries I've made it part of my routine to listen carefully to kids' answering tapes—they often contain similar not-so-secret announcements of their second-family identities.

A source of second-family reality is online communication. Teen e-mails are intensely personal and graphic. Kids, once they trust me enough, regularly bring in printouts of e-mail conversations. It opens the door to their vivid, secret dramas. For example, high school sophomore Jonathan's best friend Michael had a girlfriend, Liz. No one, except Jonathan, knew that Michael and Liz were involved with each other. (The relationship was a week old—privacy in the second family doesn't last much longer.) Jon, Michael, and Liz were toying with the idea of making it a threesome. By bringing in e-mail conversations, Jonathan was able to tell me what was going on, to help him make sense of this complicated situation. It was through reviewing these online chats that the picture slowly became clearer to Jonathan—and allowed him to think about whether he really wanted this gray-zone ménage à trois to come off.

Just about every night kids have intense arguments online, while their parents remain clueless in the next room. References may be made to all manner of experiences that are not being discussed with you. Paula was having a furious exchange with one of her friends, Angela, who had accused her of coming on to a boy that Angela herself was interested in. "Paula, of all people, with your eating disorder, *you* should know what it feels like to be lied to like this!" Not one adult, including me, realized Paula was wrestling with such a serious problem.

Other "superficial" pop culture items are deeply revealing. The magazines in my waiting room are like magnets for kids. Teens often arrive early, just to be able to leaf through back issues. They also bring in their own magazines with stories that have special meaning. Invariably, these set off discussions about their hidden feelings—crushes, school gossip, ruminations about looks. Middle-schooler Harley, an avid reader of *Teen People,* had just read an article in the waiting room about a Hollywood star with dyslexia. The story prompted Harley to open up about an embarrassing topic that she'd been hiding from her parents and me—how girls in her school would constantly disparage her for being much slower verbally than others. Harley didn't have a glam look to compensate. But worse, she couldn't mix it up in ordinary school banter.

Joey, referred for "oppositional disorder" that included tormenting classmates, had another side, which gradually emerged as he went through my magazines and demonstrated a keen eye toward style. In his school, he was one of the poorer kids. The upscale images Joey saw in the magazines made him talk about how inferior he felt to the kids that he taunted. In comparison, they all seemed to have endless resources. A superficial, pop culture magazine was my entrée into a self-conscious world hidden behind his defiant, sadistic posturing.

Music, video games, e-mail conversations, magazines—the superficial detritus of the second-family's pop culture can help you get past deceits and conceits.

TALK ABOUT TEEN'S FRIENDS AS HIS OR HER FAMILY

As mentioned in Chapter 2, during the first meeting I do a quick sociogram of a preteen's or teenager's friends. I learn friends' first names, and almost every session I refer back to find out what is going on in an adolescent's everyday life. But there is another reason: When an adolescent talks about what friends are up to, he or she is checking out whether or not it is safe to talk about his or her own private decisions. For example: Tali, 13, told me that two of her friends had engaged in oral sex. This news was a prelude to something Tali was planning—she had decided to go down on the very next boy she hooked up with, no matter who. Using friends as an entrée, we soon found ourselves in a real dialogue about *her* feelings, *her* need to keep up with everyone else. It was much easier to discuss her secret deliberations (secret from adults—just about every other kid was in on her decision) by using her friends as an introduction.

Zach told me all his friends were into gansta rap music. One of the basic themes was graffiti, and his best friend, Erik, was heavily into it. I was slow on the uptake, but Zach was telling me something: *He* was the one, not Erik, who was writing graffiti in the middle of the night. Unbeknownst to his mother, Erik snuck out just about every evening to write on public trains in train yards and on the sides of buildings. This had moved way beyond the gray zone. Discussing his friend helped me get Mom to realize the scope of his dangerous and illegal activity—before tragedy struck.

Jackie talked repeatedly about one of her friends, Emma, who had a history of cutting herself; Jackie was worried about Emma. One day, Jackie brought Emma along to our meeting. Together, we talked about ways Emma might get help for self-cutting. However, in the course of that session it became clear that what Jackie was really getting at was her own self-destructive behavior. Jackie—and it was Emma who brought this up—was secretly drinking at home and participating in porn chat rooms with older men. She was about to send out sexually explicit pictures of herself online. Her parents had absolutely no clue, and neither did I.

In each of these situations, conceptualizing friends as part of a teen's immediate family (just as I would mother, father, and siblings) unearthed significant truths behind the wall of silence.

THE TEST

As overt lying and selective omissions begin to lessen a bit—you are likely to start hearing about some of the hidden issues going on in an adolescent's life. Kids often bring up "gray-zone" material as a test to see how you will react, to check out the advice you offer, and, of course, to understand what you will do regarding parents and confidentiality.

For example, 15-year-old Jim tells me that he and a bunch of his friends have been hanging out at someone's house after school on most days. Every once in a while they drink, and nobody has found out about it. Thirteen-year-old Marcy tells me that on Friday a "rave" is going to happen. Marcy's parents think that she will just be sleeping over at a girlfriend's house that night, but Marcy and her friends are planning to sneak out and go to the all-night concert. Pat mentions that he secretly drives without a license to his ex-girlfriend's house, no matter what time of day or night, if she's having a crisis about whether or not to hurt herself.

*   *   *

When you get past the lying and learn more about ordinary danger, what then? It is a child professional's nightmare. What in the world do you do about confidentiality?

The Test

As trust begins to develop in the relationship, teens start sharing more dangerous, gray-zone information. These kinds of revelations are a test of you, asking:

- Is it safe to talk?
- Are you going to be able to handle what I tell you?
- Will you immediately tell my parents?
- Will you tell some other adult?
- Will you give me good advice?
- Do you trust my judgment, or are you going to treat me like a baby?
- Are you going to help me make a good decision about this?

7

TREATMENT UNBOUND

Creating "Flexible Confidentiality"

Momma always said, life is like a box of chocolates—you never know what you're gonna get.

—*Forrest Gump*

You can observe a lot by watching.

—*Yogi Berra*

Be careful what you wish for. Sometimes you wish you didn't know; you would have preferred living with the lies, rather than the gray zone of an adolescent's life. Like me, you find out that the 12-year-old *you* see has been regularly snorting Ritalin or heroin after school in friends' empty houses. Or, you learn that *your* 13-year-old client wants to get his tongue pierced, without his parents' knowledge. Or, the 14-year-old in treatment with *you* is talking about having lots of unprotected sex. Or, you discover from *your* high school junior how he sneaks out night after night without anyone in his house knowing. Or, you hear from a high school senior about plans to spend weekend nights in abandoned buildings trying out the life of anarchists and squatters.

What do you do with the information? Shouldn't parents automatically know? Isn't it your professional responsibility? Yet, isn't it part of your role to maintain confidentiality?

Kids Lie—We Lie

It is not clear what child professionals ought to do with gray zone information. Take a moment to consider the pressures that encourage adults who treat teens to omit information or simply lie to parents. It is amazing to me how little we discuss this complex professional issue.

Start with the continued emphasis on a boundaried container. Nothing except for *imminent* danger needs to be shared with parents. This prohibition is ingrained, reinforced by HIPAA regulations—a prohibition that might have made sense when kids were petting in parked cars, not being sexually active in an era of AIDS.

Ratchet things up a bit. When an adolescent begins treatment, many parents feel they've handed their child over to you. They may not want to know what is really going on. The growing pains, the worries, the acting out are now *your* responsibility. Your role has become one of *in loco parentis*.

Now add clinical theory. For much of the past century a strong undertone of distrust (especially toward mothers) existed. Mothers and fathers—despite growing biological evidence—are the ones who "cause" difficulties in the kids we see. Why trust in the very people who created the problems for your client in the first place?

Then consider a final force that shuts up child professionals: Adolescents feel a sense of *entitlement* to privacy. Privacy is an integral right, along with many rights that are, indeed, essential—the right not to be abused, the right to be treated respectfully, the right to question adults, and the right to be listened to, among others. Ask teenagers, as I have, and you will hear yet another right—a sense of entitlement to an adolescence unfettered by any adult intrusion.

These forces can create a therapy relationship that exists far away from significant adults in kids' lives. The last thing teens need is a counselor who is afraid to share truths that might narrow the gap between kids and adults, yet that is precisely the conundrum therapists are caught in. Gray-zone behavior practically screams out for honesty, yet openness may betray a client, may trigger harsh parental reactions and complex administrative or legal issues.

This is why I begin treatment reversing figure and ground: "Tell me what you *don't* want me to share." This is why I try to see past kids' façade early on, why I set my threshold for concern at a much lower level than "immediate danger." The earlier I can open the boundaries of treatment without betraying a child's trust, the less lying by omission I do with a teen's parents. It is a difficult balancing act: *how to guarantee privacy as you keep watch over an often dangerous teen world, yet how to gain trust if kids believe you are monitoring their behavior.* This is *the* challenge of working with teens today, living ever at the edge. Unless the balance is continuously addressed—with kids, with parents, with oneself—the helping relationship is structurally flawed. We need ways to deal with this dilemma; we need ways to create "flexible confidentiality" that brings kids and parents closer.

CONFIDENTIALITY FOR KIDS: ENTITLEMENT OR PRIVILEGE?

For years I have suggested that teens are not entitled to unconditional privacy at home, they must earn it. This goes for confidentiality in treatment, too. Think of professional confidentiality as an envelope that expands as a teen handles responsibilities. The more a child gains the trust of his parents and me, the more privacy I can promise in our relationship. After all, when kids first present, it is usually for serious reasons. At the same time, I know very little; I have almost no way to trust his or her safety enough to guarantee absolute privacy.

Fifteen-year-old Malcolm was sent to me because he was cutting school, would stay out for entire evenings and not come home on weekends. He carried around a huge reserve of rage, occasionally erupting toward his parents and teachers. I didn't know, and neither did his parents, who Malcolm's friends were, what his fantasies were about, what his everyday life was like. I had no idea how Malcolm actually spent his time behind that closed door, no way of knowing what world he was into, what his nocturnal gray-zone activities were—sex, drugs, drinking, other illegal behaviors? How could I guarantee Malcolm *carte blanche* privacy without knowing a single real detail about his life?

Ava was an extremely moody girl who was getting into fights with adults and friends across the board. Neither, her mother nor I, knew any of her buddies, how she spent her afternoons while Mom worked or what interests she had. We had no idea whether she was actively involved in drugs or sex. We didn't know what she did behind that façade at home or when she was out. Was she safe or was she in deeper danger than anyone realized? Ava hadn't revealed much of this to previous therapists; she tenaciously guarded her unfettered freedom.

The idea that from the start Malcolm or Ava ought to be entitled to absolute confidentiality is a mistake. Behind the "wall of silence" exists an unknown world. Yet, how can the work proceed without guaranteeing some degree of what kids (and professional ethics) consider an entitlement? The answer is what I call "flexible confidentiality."

Flexible Confidentiality

Remember what I say to clients in the first session: "Tell me what you *don't* want me to reveal to anyone." Rather than promising that all topics are confidential, I continue, *"We'll talk about what you don't want me to say, and we'll figure out how to handle it together."* To this, I add the following reassurance: *"I'll never mention anything to your parents before you and I talk it over, unless I believe . . . and here's the part you already know . . . that you or someone else is in immediate danger."*

How do kids react to this turn of events? Some ask, "Why do you have to say *anything* to my parents?" My answer is "Well, I'm also here to help your parents be more effective with you. And that's in your interest. The better they feel about the way they are with you, the more privileges you're going to end up with."

In a sense, the situation is on turned its head—going from "Everything except danger will be kept private" to *"Nothing* is private unless you tell me it is—and even then, we'll need to talk about it." You might think that adolescents would pull back immediately, thinking "I'm not telling anything to this 'shrink.' " In my experience, however, they usually feel the opposite. My commitment to their parents, not just them, clearly states that the adults also need to change. It is a welcome discovery if kids have been the focus of blame. To most teens, this is worth my offer of flexible confidentiality.

Earl, 18, had just finished his first term of college in a small southern school, a miserable experience. In our sessions, he went into a litany of details about life in the dorm. Everything was topsy-turvy—breakfast was lunch, lunch was dinner, dinner might be wolfing down food at three in the morning. Marijuana was instantly accessible. Kids binge drank huge amounts of liquor. One of the two town bars featured low-cost alcohol, just for students. Students cut classes much of the time, and it didn't seem to matter to anyone. Now, out of all this, the one thing Earl didn't want his parents to know was that he smoked pot. Earl was in no immediate danger, but how could his parents and he discuss college plans without getting into the specific details about his college activities?

Mark, 14, was also not in immediate danger, but was profoundly isolated, a loner who had no connections with other children. The phone never rang. His parents were unable to name one classmate they could call a friend. Mark spent huge blocks of time by himself, secretly living in a pornographic, violent fantasy world inhabited by unknown kids and adults in cyberspace. Mark described these activities to me, but said, "My parents don't know about this stuff. I don't want you to say anything to them—they'll just think I'm wasting my time or that I'm crazy." But, in fact, Mark's parents were being driven crazy with worry, and their constant intrusions to monitor his well-being (searching his room, unsuccessfully trying to track his computer activities), only caused him to withdraw further.

Fifteen-year-old Zoe told me, "Listen, just about every kid in my grade has been getting drunk every weekend since we were in eighth grade. There are a lot of empty houses in this town. It isn't a big deal, it happens all the time. But I don't want you to mention this to my mother—everything else is OK, but not this!" We discussed her drinking in detail, enough for me to get a sense that although Zoe wasn't in immediate danger, the specifics of her weekend activities were critical for Mom to know in order to understand what kind of privileges made sense for her daughter.

Despite my announcement that material from our work might also help their parents become more attuned, these kids opened up to me. How could this be? As I mentioned in Chapter 2, there are several reasons: Once treatment begins, many teens simply forget our "deal." Others could care less. They believe their parents—caught up in their own worlds of divorce, dislocation, addiction, or financial pressures—don't have real power, anyway. So, it doesn't *matter* what they know. Or kids feel I'm not going to bother to say much, anyway. Or, being kids, they're so embroiled in the events of that particular week, adults are irrelevant, a distant speck on the horizon of adolescent life. Or, the few teens who still *do* unconsciously want to be "caught" feel relieved that their descent into the second family might be slowed down a bit.

The majority of kids don't feel threatened by flexible confidentiality. When they reserve their right to privacy about specific information, these areas become a primary focus of our discussions. The reasons for not telling parents, our differences of opinion, and their knowledge that I'm working to "fix" their parents, too, become a central part of the relationship.

Earl and I spent two meetings imagining whether his recently separated parents would really be all that stunned about his smoking marijuana. Finally, he decided they wouldn't be and we could focus on the real issue—leaving home when his mom and dad were still embroiled in an unresolved custody battle over his brother.

Mark and I talked a lot about his cyberworlds, so much so that after many meetings it became normalized enough that he no longer even cared whether they knew. Zoe, on the other hand, refused to budge. She continued to insist that her weekend activities remain with me. However, in the process, Zoe slowly began to hear my concerns about her drinking, and one night let her mother "discover" it by vomiting all over the house.

It's uncomfortable to argue about confidentiality. But the traction created in our relationship and at home opens up endless material.

PARENTS' RIGHTS

Since I do not define confidentiality primarily in terms of immediate danger, I focus a lot on the gray zone: *ordinary 21st-century teen life*. What must parents know to achieve a greater balance between empathy and expectations—in ways that keep kids safe and help them to grow? I want parents to become effective. I believe they are more important to change than whatever happens in the consulting room.

To do this, kids know from early on that I will be having infrequent, but regular, contact with their parent(s). This is not a secret. What I don't tell kids is the underlying rationale: *I hope an adolescent will sense a growing adult presence in his or her life*. I want her to "get" that her parents may become smarter and more tuned in, that we adults are all trying to grasp the complexities of the second family, the difficult decisions that must be made daily. Over time, then, I hope kids will feel held by the adults at home, not just by the second family out there.

Talking to Parents—without Breaking Confidentiality: Five Guidelines

TEMPERAMENT MATTERS

The more I understand a teen's temperament, the more I share that understanding with mothers and fathers. Many have already spoken with various mental health practitioners, most of whom are well trained and well intentioned. Nevertheless, parents often arrive feeling guilt-ridden for what has gone wrong with their kids. Despite extensive research over the past two decades, few professionals validate the temperamental reality of kids, the specific, idiosyncratic challenges parent have faced from the beginning.

An alliance with a mother or father is profoundly strengthened by *sharing* your experience of their adolescent's temperament: The teen who had always been shy, who now has terrible fears entering new peer groups; another who has been fiercely tenacious from the time she was a toddler, and who is no less stubborn as a teenager;

another who was always more active than others, and now can't possibly be reined in; another whose attention was so laser-focused that his parents needed to repeat themselves 10 times, a trait exponentially aggravated during the attentionally challenged teen years.

By sharing observations about a child's hard-wiring, I let parents know I understand what they've been up against. This is often an "Aha!" experience: *"Somebody finally gets who I've had to deal with from the start."* They feel less shamed; it's not *all* their fault. In fact, given the chronicity of the challenge, many parents actually handle matters better than they ever realized. Empathic understanding of temperament creates a *"readiness for change"* (see my earlier book *Getting Through to Difficult Kids and Parents*, 2001), which helps parents follow your directives.

Warren, 13½, mentioned a ridiculous remark he made to another kid in school, who then ignored him. I asked, "I know you feel bad. But, what did you expect this kid to say?" Warren replied, "I just wanted an answer from him." We went round and round. This was a lifelong characteristic of Warren's. He would become concrete, unable to grasp what might be going on in another person. This stubbornness was exactly what his parents experienced every day of his life. Warren dug himself into an unmovable position, which triggered their impatience until everybody flew into near-physical rages. When Mom and Dad were able to hear that I *got it*, that I understood their son's maddening concreteness— "Aha! This guy knows first-hand what it's been like with our kid. We love him, but he's so stubborn and dense we could scream!"— they also heard what Warren needed from them.

Ian, 15, was one of the most adept con artists I ever met. He could spin such a yarn, tell such a story, that almost every adult would believe anything he said. Ian was basically a good-hearted kid—with a silver tongue that got him into more trouble than it got him out of. If Ian showed up late for a session, he almost had me buying his tale that the dog ate his homework. Or he had been saving some person's life, so he couldn't get to my office on time. Given my views on flexible confidentiality, I would describe to Dad frustrating exchanges with Ian, much to his delight and growing belief that I was not just another parent-bashing professional. A veteran of Ian's con-artistry since the preschool years, he believed that some adult was finally on the same page with him.

With Angelina's parents I shared the following from our individual meetings: "I can't believe how single-minded your daughter is. When she wants something, she won't stop." Angelina was the girl who insisted on reading my notes. I told her more than once, "You can't read these because they have other peoples' names in them." It was all I could do to prevent her from grabbing the notebook out of my hand. My description to Angelina's parents was invaluable at creating traction. They had been dealing with her tenacity since toddlerhood. Yet most professionals implied that Mom, especially, had caused it all—spoiling her child, turning her daughter into a tyrant.

This is an easy way to establish a connection, sharing information about temperamental characteristics with parents. It creates a readiness for change, especially regarding the childrearing strategies discussed in Chapter 8. It is easy because kids obviously don't care much whether you discuss their temperament. How, though, does one share more private matters without losing teens' trust?

Thinking in terms of flexible confidentiality, there are four other ways to bring up difficult issues with parents, while protecting the treatment relationship.

GENERALLY SPEAKING

Introducing a topic in general terms, without getting into details, helps parents focus on what really matters. Most adults don't see the big picture of teen life. Parents are often narrowly stuck on a particular issue, such as the messy room, bad-influence friends, a specific drug, sex, grades, or vague concerns about "the future." Bringing up a topic in general helps them learn about important details *now*, without your having to break confidentiality.

For example, I met with Earl's separated parents, the late adolescent who had returned home depressed from his first year of college. If you remember, I was absolutely "forbidden" to say anything about his smoking pot. Earl's parents cooperated by being entirely focused on his academic performance—the tendency for Earl to be "lazy" and "easily distracted." Their arguments about his character and motivation were understandable, but way off the mark.

When we met, I asked them, as I have many other parents of freshman college kids: "What do you imagine dorm life is like these days?" This general question was a way to help Mom and Dad picture the past year, to discover for *themselves* what their son had told me *not* to say. Reflecting on the nitty-gritty details of college life triggered memories of their own chaotic undergraduate experiences: staying up forever; day/night cycles turned upside down; the sex, drugs, and alcohol scene, especially when big-name rock bands gave concerts. After painting a detailed picture about their own lives, it was a natural step for Dad to ask Earl about alcohol and pot. Not surprisingly (the commercials are right—parents don't talk enough to kids), Earl began to 'fess up. Mom and Dad "got" what a rough ride 21st-century dorm life can be. They realized it was still necessary to be involved with Earl in an ongoing way: more phone calls and e-mails, helping to anchor Earl's chaotic routines: Dad would call mornings, just to "chat" and get the day started; Mom helped him negotiate educational support possibilities, and so on. I never broke Earl's confidentiality. Just by introducing the general issue of "dorm life," I didn't need to. Earl was greatly relieved. Paradoxically, the more his parents knew, the more grown-up he felt. A year later they ended up deciding to reconcile. But, soon after this change in their stance toward Earl and some focused family sessions (see Chapter 9) Earl's worries about them had already lessened.

EYES WIDE SHUT: GETTING PARENTS TO SEE

Parents often don't see what is right in front of them. They are unwilling to open their eyes and notice the small but highly revealing details. Confused, afraid or oblivious, their actions typically fail. In addition, their vision is blurred about teen realities *now*: They forget their own adolescent years and what it felt like—or, just the opposite— they incorrectly assume that being a teen today is exactly the same as it was for them. Like the title of that Tom Cruise and Nicole Kidman movie, they live with their *Eyes Wide Shut*.

Fourteen-year-old Jean was drinking and smoking at weekend parties and occasionally on weekday afternoons. No adult had noticed a thing, except that she was becoming less motivated in school and had less passion for her usual interests. We were in the gray zone. At some point Jean's mother needed to open her eyes, or else Jean was in danger of drifting further into the second family and possible addiction. I brought up the subject without saying much at all: "What do you actually see when Jean comes home?"

This specific question made Mom take notice next time. When Jean came home she looked spacey, rushed to get something to eat, didn't kiss Mom goodnight, and for several days afterwards couldn't focus on her work. Without my saying a word about specifics, Mom began to ask Jean directly, "Are you OK? Where did you just come from? Let's talk for a while." A couple of weeks later, alcohol and pot smoking were open for discussion. Jean was still downplaying her real activities, but at least Mom had gotten the issue on the table—without my needing to wait for "immediate danger" to develop.

Another client, Myles, a 15-year-old high school sophomore, was moving toward unprotected sex with his sexually experienced senior girlfriend, Patti, who'd had many partners—some with extremely high-risk backgrounds. Myles was prone to crippling self-doubt about his adequacy in most every area. Sex was a way to counter self-doubt. But, Patti? He wasn't sure how he felt about her, and he was asking no adult for input except me. His mother, Dawn, needed to see more. So I said to her, "When Patti is around, what do you think? Is his door open or closed?" She replied that the door was often closed. I said, "OK, what might that mean?" I said nothing else. But the next time Dawn noticed the closed door, she was unable to ignore it. At first she said to herself, "No, he's too much of a baby and a whiny mess at that. I don't think they're even close to anything serious." But, then, she added, "Kids do get older; and that door is closed a lot."

This was a turning point: Dawn began to see that, despite his psychological vulnerabilities, Myles was, indeed, growing up.

Then, *she* started hesitatingly talking to him about sex; surprisingly, Myles opened up just a tiny bit. Dawn got to know Patti better and began talking to her as a young woman. Mom's notions about her little boy shifted; she finally saw he was at the edge of becoming a sexually active young adult, out there in the world of girls. The more Dawn could see the realities, the more she could offer Myles some guidance about whether this time and this girlfriend should be his first time sexually, especially if Patti refused HIV testing. It was amazing to watch them go from no discussion at all to ones that included graphic details. Patti agreed, and tested negative. But, because of his mixed feelings, Myles held off on sex (meaning intercourse) with her. Two years and two girlfriends later it happened for Myles, in a way and with someone that felt right to him.

GET PARENTS TO THINK THE UNTHINKABLE

Most mothers and fathers find it impossible to imagine kids involved in the behaviors they are engaging in, especially the kinds of raunchy, at-the-edge decisions kids make without blinking an eye. Adults may realize it at some level, but don't actually know it. Christopher Bollas, the relational psychologist, coined a phrase that describes this psychic phenomenon. He calls it "the unthought known" (Shadow of the Object, 1987). We *know,* but we don't really think about it and don't name it.

Part of your job is to get parents to put into words "unthought knowns" about their kids. Without divulging confidences say, "It's unimaginable, but I want you to try to think about your child differently." You don't have to be specific about what a client has shared with you; rather you stretch parents' narrow concept of their child toward a fuller, though certainly more uncomfortable, perception. It is what they knew, but didn't want to know.

Twelve-year-old Joanna wasn't able to keep up with her friends' sophisticated verbal give-and-take. In the second family there is a lot of dissing and lightning-fast repartee. When a child cannot keep pace, it's hard to fit in. Joanna knew her problem and was disappearing into a shell of self-consciousness. Joanna told me, "Everybody kids around, and I don't know what to say. By the time I think of something, they're already on to the next thing. But I'm too embarrassed to say anything—and you can't tell anybody either, especially my parents," she cried to me. "I have better friends on TV than in my life."

Joanna's parents are articulate individuals. Joanna's younger sister was also quick-witted. It may not seem like much, but to this mother and father it was unthinkable that their older child could- n't keep up. I told them, "When Joanna is with other kids, just pay attention. As Yogi Berra said, 'You can observe a lot by watching.' " The unthinkable, that Joanna was the only one in their family who couldn't engage in quick conversation, slowly became clear. Once I pushed them to recognize the unthought known, it became starkly apparent without my having to say more. This was an important step toward change—psychoeducational testing followed. Over time they began to see Joanna more clearly, deal with their disappointment, and get her the language remediation she really needed. An actual social life (with all its dangers) now became the new concern.

With 16-year-old Paul the unthinkable concerned money, spe- cifically how he was getting it. Paul was an "anarchist" who lived in working-class suburbia. He was at serious odds with most of the mainstream kids and the school's administrative hierarchy. At home he was sullen, a black hole to his mother and aunt. Paul's biggest passion was being an aficionado of eBay. Occasionally, FedEx packages would show up at the door. A family of modest means, his mother didn't know where the money was coming from to buy this stuff. But the truth was right in front of their eyes— Paul regularly took tiny amounts of cash from various family mem- bers in one way or another. Hearing her concerns (though Paul told me nothing about his activities, either), I encouraged Mom to think the unthinkable: "Just stay aware. That's all you need to do." Indeed, it *was* all mom needed to do. She began to thoroughly check ATM statements, as well as track dollar bills in wallets and change left out around the house. Very soon, the reality she had been sensing became clear. Mom had known all along, but again, it had remained the unthought known.

Fifteen-year-old Alex is gay and had not told his parents; everyone in his world was aware of this except them. Alex forbade me from discussing this—a request I, of course, honored. Alex was fearful about telling his parents, who are from a conservative, fundamentalist background. At the same time, he was deeply contemptuous about their "stupidity." Alex's fierce contempt and shame pushed him to take risks that were clearly in the gray zone of danger—binge drinking, baiting the toughest kids at school, constant fighting that left him open to revenge. Despite their conservative roots, Alex's *mother and father knew the reality, but did not know.* I needed to keep his trust, yet do something that would break this paralysis.

When I met with them, I said: "I want you to watch your son as if you were seeing him for the first time. What are his interests? Whom does he hang out with? Who are his friends? Pay attention, and open your mind up to whatever the possibilities may be." That was the beginning of Alex's very slow coming-out. Without saying a word to Alex or me, his mother and father gradually began to accept Alex's male friends—one of whom was, in fact, his boyfriend. My encouragement to observe, allowed them to, at least slowly, consider the unthinkable. The more open they were (though nothing was ever concretely mentioned about Alex's sexual orientation), the less risky Alex's acting out became.

HOW TO HELP PARENTS TALK ABOUT IMPOSSIBLE TOPICS

It is the 21st century. And those annoying public service advertisements are true—many parents still can't start conversations with kids about dicey subjects. Parents often feel like they're not the real experts. After all, schools now deal with sex, drug, and "life issues," starting in the midelementary grades; television brings up every difficult subject imaginable. In a way, adults are both off the hook and overpowered by the information explosion all around. In addition, many parents will not bring up sex, drugs, or drinking for fear of "putting ideas into a teen's head." Parents think that as soon as it's mentioned, their impressionable child will say, "Gee, I never thought of that." Just the opposite is true; even preteen kids are bombarded everyday with messages—porn e-mail, graphic magazines, edgy TV shows (*Sex and the City* is practically required viewing for many youngsters—syndicated reruns have ensured this for another decade), graphic song lyrics, anime, violent video games, adult movies on demand—it is an endless, lurid, in-your-face world. Most kids are insulted that we believe they're so suggestible, or that parental words are more powerful than the ordinary realities they face.

One teenage boy enlightened me about this issue. My own children were just approaching that online age, and I was particularly interested in his remarks. "How should parents handle the Web?" I asked, trying to sound neutral. He said, "I know you're worried about your own kids, and you can put all kinds of parental controls and filters on the computer. But you're gonna have to be prepared that just about everything will get through anyway. So, whether you want to or not, you need to talk to them about porn." Nice. An early adolescent encouraging *me* to talk about this subject with my own children.

Many parents complain endlessly about second-family behavior, but never actually broach issues with their teens. At the risk of sounding like that generic TV spot, they need to be encouraged to do so. For example, 15-year-old Jon kept his bedroom *padlocked*, not particularly unusual these days, I learn from my lectures around the country. It seemed unnecessary, since his single father, Anthony, was far from being oppressive. On top of this "heavy-metal" signal, Jon drew intense artwork that looked as if it was informed by hallucinogens. In fact, Anthony was pretty sure Jon smoked pot and maybe even took acid in the house—which I knew to be correct. But for the reasons listed earlier, this sophisticated, savvy parent just could not see his way toward asking his son about any of this. "I'm afraid he'll think that I don't trust him and that I think he's a baby." I urged Anthony to take a chance—bring up the subject, at least pot smoking, just to show Jon he wasn't completely clueless.

When Anthony was finally able to take the plunge, Jon had a typical teen reaction. First, he was outraged: "How *dare* you question me!" Second, he immediately saw his father as less "stupid," and not so clueless as to miss what was patently obvious to him and all his friends. This opening led to discussions in which Anthony talked about his own "Woodstock-generation" past. No illusions here—Jon did not entirely give up smoking, although his LSD use ended. However, he cut marijuana down enough that he was able to use his newfound mental energy to develop a passion— painting! The change process began at the exact moment Jon's dad swallowed hard and spoke to him. Without my breaking confidentiality, Jon reevaluated his rock-solid belief that Dad was just another dumb adult he could get over on.

Fourteen-year-old Meredith was a brightly lit neon sign of sexuality and substance use—the clothing she wore, the kids she hung around with, the stores and neighborhoods she frequented. But her single mother, Courtney, like many parents, had never been able to initiate a real conversation with her daughter about any graphic details of sex. She was embarrassed. Courtney did not ask, did not want to know; yet she was worried down to her bones. How far had Meredith gone? What were her attitudes about sex? Did she want to sleep with the boy she was spending so much time with? Did they smoke up together? I knew the answers to most of these questions, but Meredith wanted a wall around her confidences. Unfortunately, Mom said nothing, choosing to leave all such concerns up to me, the media, the peer group, and the school. Courtney needed to be pushed to talk to her daughter.

Courtney and I role-played "discussing tough stuff." For weeks our practice dialogues, which included her concerns about Meredith's obvious sexuality, did not change a thing on the home front. Then one night, seemingly out of nowhere, Mom said to her daughter: "A new CD, $17; a spring dress, $45, a heart-to-heart talk with your daughter—priceless! . . . So are you thinking about sex with Deon?" Meredith laughed despite herself and then immediately ran screaming, out of the room. But the ice was broken. After a week of silence mom *demanded* a conversation, or no date that weekend. Finally, they had several hesitant, heart-to-hearts about how the world is different now: Mom recalled her own interest in boys—how provocatively she had once dressed herself, showing Meredith some of her vintage outfits; they discussed what sex meant back then and what "hooking up" means now.

With my encouragement during our individual meetings, Meredith began to talk to Mom a little more about decisions she had to make at every middle school party. These were at once much starker and more casual than her mother had ever realized: whether to give a guy head, not whether to make out; whether to hook up with boys *and* girls, not just boys; whether to binge drink hard liquor, not just have a beer—and many other decisions Mom never considered before the end of high school. Mother and daughter started filling in the blanks between them. There was no dramatic change in Meredith's flamboyant presentation; she was still sexually provocative and willing to experiment at the edges. But the edge was slightly closer to home, her drift out to the second family a little less dramatic. Casual hooking up in groups became less automatic. With Mom's input, Meredith began a new journey—experiencing her sexuality as a force she had some control over, rather than a force that controlled her.

Beyond the Gray Zone and into Danger

These ways to convey information to parents without breaking confidentiality are useful in the gray zone of teen life. Often, however, working with adolescents invariably means being drawn into truly dangerous situations. You no longer have freedom to make the same subtle judgment calls. *When a child is involved in imminent danger, you must act.* This is a reason therapists ought not see too many teens at once. Springtime is particularly tough; the months of February to May are terribly trying. At least one or two of my teen clients are guaranteed to keep me at the edge of my seat. Ultimately, adolescents engaging in risky business warrants breaking confidentiality.

"Risky business" I mean in the traditional sense: (1) A teenager is in immediate danger—it could well be a matter of life or death; (2) a dangerous event has already occurred that must be shared; or (3) your client talks to you about something that is going to happen and you feel that that it is a harmful decision.

Many examples come to mind, some I have mentioned earlier. A 13-year-old boy talked to me about having had sex for the first time. Not only was he 13, but the incident happened when he was drunk, the sex was unprotected, and he planned on more the next weekend. A 16-year-old was involved in 100-mph drag races on abandoned stretches of road. A 13-year-old girl had a secret ruminative disorder, focusing on "accidents" that could happen to her or her family. The talk took an even more serious turn as she began describing her ability to telepathically communicate with others. A 14-year-old girl suddenly showed me tracks of scars she'd secretly carved into her leg. In many situations, especially with volatile or fragile teens, there is simply no room to postpone. All bets are off, and parents or other adults need to be told. The legal or ethical consequences are a concern for anyone who takes on tough kids.

Nevertheless, it is still very difficult to "pull the plug," and for good reason: We worry that it might make matters worse. Regardless of whether your action was absolutely necessary, it is often a deathblow to the relationship. You've spent months, perhaps years, gaining trust, and now one phone call may destroy it all. The upshot is that by acting ethically, you might end up destroying the relationship.

This irreparable rupture is a key reason for getting parents to open their eyes before it is too late, and it is a key reason to push your client to start sharing more with parents before you'll be forced to.

For example, Todd, a 15-year-old boy, had been sneaking out of his house at 2:00 in the morning to roam the streets with his posse of friends. When their activities became clearly dangerous—getting into knife fights, graffiti in frighteningly high places—I had to challenge the privacy of our relationship. His dad took appropriate action, but what I had to reveal was so serious, I lost Todd's trust. He would never talk to me again.

A 15-year-old girl, Ginny, told me about going on a three-day cocaine binge and sleeping with several boys in just as many days. As soon as I found out about it, I needed to inform her parents. It had to be done, but our work was over.

When behavior is serious enough for hospitalization or a structured program, other professionals enter. Once again, the relationship may be lost. I was seeing a 16-year-old boy who had been smoking pot on and off; he'd been in the gray zone for a while. But when he moved into smoking heroin, there was no holding back from bringing it to his parent's attention. Within a week he was evaluated for drug use and admitted to a substance abuse program. That was the last I saw him in ongoing therapy.

Must it always end this way? When you can't get parents to notice, see, or think the unthinkable—how can you act on an imminent danger without breaking trust?

Getting Kids to Spill the Beans

If danger must be addressed, begin with giving teens a chance to tell parents themselves. If there is time, push kids to be frank about the dangerous behavior they believe their parents are going to "freak out" about. There are three ways to handle this.

SET A TIME LIMIT TO SPEAK TO PARENTS

With adolescents it is usually essential to impose a time limit. Many teens, like younger children, have a poor concept of time. Their estimates are completely off, and weeks simply slip through their fingers. Kids often have undeveloped executive functioning. It sounds harsh, but working with teens is like working with the attentionally challenged, or, worse, with cases of early-onset Alzheimer's: The moment adolescents leave your presence, many have totally forgotten what was discussed or what you just told them. The issue may seem extremely serious and one *we* think would be incredibly important—telling parents about brushes with police, first-time sex, hard drugs, or near-death experiences. Yet even non-resistant teens are likely to forget the moment they reach the street—or even sooner.

Most avoid being candid to adults about danger, *unless they believe the situation will not be allowed to drag on indefinitely*. Without time limits, a self-perpetuating cycle sets in: The riskier the behavior—the more lying is a necessity—the more lying occurs, the further teens move into the orbit of the second family; the more into the second family they are, the more distant kids feel from parents, and the less conflicted they feel about continuing to lie.

Teens feel omnipotent, and are great at forgetting the distant world of consequences. They excel at putting off, dissembling, relying on the wall of silence to protect. And, very often, they are *not* afraid of your reaction, they are *not* afraid of their parents' reaction, they are *not* afraid of the school's reaction. The only concern that stays on their screen is the possibility of losing access to the second family.

OFFER A LIMITED CHOICE FOR "WHEN"

With so much on the line, borrow from the work of hypnotherapist Milton Erickson and offer a "limited choice." Child development researchers have demonstrated the effectiveness of offering limited choices to difficult three-year-olds. Like toddlers, adolescents are among the most tenacious human beings. When cornered, they need the combined structure *and* autonomy of a limited choice: "Tell your parents this week or next, today or tomorrow," depending on the degree of danger. As long as you can live with either decision a teen makes, a limited choice preserves a sense of autonomy and pushes the process forward.

CREATE CONSEQUENCES IF A TEEN CHOOSES NOT
TO MOVE TOWARD OPENNESS

Adolescents need to know that inaction will lead to a consequence ("If you can't tell your parents, then *I'll* have to.") As a progressive psychologist, it was hard for me to grasp that many kids might only respond to consequences. But I've listened to countless 12–16-year-olds say the one thing that gets through to them is the idea of a concrete response. Kids in danger need to feel the possibility of consequences, *if for no other reason than to help them remember.*

Here are some examples using these three guidelines to help kids spill the beans:

For weeks Chris had been setting up an online date with a girl (an increasingly "ordinary" phenomenon). He'd met this stranger in a "bipolar" chat room (yes, you read this correctly). Since for logistical reasons the date would not happen for a month, I decided a couple of weeks would be a workable time limit. I said to Chris, "Over the next three weeks, we're going to have to figure out some way you can talk to one of your parents about what you're planning. I don't care which one. Otherwise, as much as I don't want to, I'll have to do it myself. I'd rather it come from you." Chris was outraged. After his initial reaction, though, we began to discuss whether it made sense to talk to his mother or father. Chris thought that his mom was too hysterical (having a bipolar disorder herself) and would tell other mothers. Therefore, he promised to talk to his dad, Al, who was an expert about computers. We went over scenarios about when it would be best to approach his father and role-played how he would say his piece.

Promises, role playing and advice notwithstanding, Chris hardly rushed into anything. In fact, he barely remembered any of our interactions, registering a blank look when I'd remind him in following meetings. Almost two weeks went by; I was at the edge of my seat. A day before the deadline, he approached his dad. (These cliffhangers are part of why adults who work with teens are so stressed out.) Al was visibly relieved that Chris had come to him, and was smart enough not to get too crazed about his son's plan. He didn't immediately forbid it, which would only have made Chris more determined. Dad used his computer expertise to learn more about the girl. They found out where she lived and were even able to learn something about her background, which included several arrests. The father then offered to accompany Chris to the motel and remain somewhere in the background; Dad was going out on a limb, but he felt it would never come to that. And it didn't. Somewhere in the course of opening this up, it became clear, even to Chris, that the meeting was "probably not the best idea." In the end, after all the fireworks, getting Chris to talk to his father helped create greater traction and trust between them.

Matthew was a 17-year-old boy who was arranging to buy a

motorcycle with a sidecar for ridiculously little money—from people he didn't know at all *and* behind his parent's back. Here's how some of our discussions went:

MATT: I'm really making headway. But you can't say anything to my parents, you know they won't let me.

THERAPIST: I can't promise I won't say anything ever. I need to hear more of the details. How in the world will you get certification of ownership? You're underage.

MATT: That's easy. There are plenty of places you can get fake IDs.

THERAPIST: Knowing your parents, do you think you stand a better chance of pulling off this whole charade without their involvement or if you talk it over with them beforehand? Weren't they discussing an old used car for your 18th birthday?

MATT: Yeah, they'll be upset, but I don't want that old car. It's not cool enough.

THERAPIST: So you want to be the host, who can impress *and* take people back and forth.

MATT: Yeah, I'll drive my best friends around. I really like that. I'll fix the side-car up and make it real comfortable."

[A note: When Matt first started seeing me, he had an anxiety disorder. He was improving somewhat in that regard and was now making a lot of friends. Matt is an example of a teen who, as he gets better, *gets into more trouble*. In an effort to enhance his new social standing, he was planning to develop a "second family cycle service," as well as perhaps joining the local chapter of the Hell's Angels—quite a development for a once anxious, ruminative, hypochondriacal young adolescent.]

THERAPIST: I get the picture, and I'm a little envious. But, it also worries me. Suppose something happens on the way back. You'll have no insurance.

MATT: C'mon, what can happen?

THERAPIST: Your parents will absolutely flip and rightfully so, because it's not only dangerous, it's illegal. I really want you to have transportation, but not this way. They'll never trust you again, and they probably won't trust me either.

MATT: Why should I care about that? They don't trust me anyway.

THERAPIST: Are you sure? Think about all the privileges you've gotten during the last year. [At this point, Mathew, who was a consummate negotiator, started realizing that his parent's anger could well trigger the loss of privileges he already had.] Look, how about a month? If you or we haven't figured out a way to approach your parents, then I'll absolutely have to tell them. I'm not going to have any choice."

Matt got really quiet, and then tried to change the subject.

THERAPIST: No, Matt, I really mean it. I'll have no choice if we don't figure this out together.

MATT: OK, OK. I'll do something.

He walked out extremely mad at me—predictably, though, he forgot our discussion three seconds later.

For two weeks Matt continued to hide the whole business and feverishly make arrangements for his deal. As he and I went back and forth, I kept hitting on one thing that seemed to make a dent, the insurance issue. He would be driving the motorcycle back without insurance, and he was savvy enough to know that this could get his family into deep financial and legal trouble. Finally, Matt realized that the loss of privileges at home would cancel the gain in second family stature. He *did* need to bring them in on it. So he told his father, Mike. Dad exploded, just as Matt had anticipated. But after Mike settled down, they talked a lot about the issue of purchasing a motorcycle from a stranger. Then they struck a deal: Matt and his dad bought an old motorcycle for a couple of hundred dollars, one they could rebuild together, almost from scratch. Using our confidentiality as a consequence, Matt came back from the brink, to a far less dangerous place.

Here is an example that did not turn out as well:

Sixteen-year-old Roberta had been smoking marijuana pretty heavily. She had given up her favorite sport, lacrosse, and although she had once been a good student, her grades were slipping fast. Roberta's phone answering machine message was provocative, and spelled out to anyone who knew a thing about pot that she was "into the life." All the signals told me I was right to be increasingly concerned, and that something needed to be said.

I confronted Roberta, telling her that she had to speak to her father or mother, who were in the process of divorcing, each having already found a new partner. Given the quickly changing family configuration, I gave her a few weeks to do so. Roberta complied, but she was so skillful at talking around things and had developed such a veneer, she was able to minimize the amount she was smoking and exploit the different views her mother and father had on the issue. She made them a promise that she would smoke only once or twice a month, if at all. I later found out she never had any intention of going along with that promise. As Roberta continued to lie to me, and in various ways wasn't sticking to our agreement, I realized she was as deeply entrenched as ever.

This time I told Roberta she had three days to talk to both her parents—otherwise we'd have a family session. The last thing she wanted was to deal with her already short-tempered parents together. Roberta was furious; she lost her cool, and walked out on our session. But I gave her no choice. Strangely enough, she decided to come clean with her mother, Mary Beth, although she had often told me how "crazy" her mom got. I think, in fact, it was a strategically smart move; Mary Beth was so pleased she had been *right* that she didn't explode. Unfortunately, her mother took such a reasonable attitude Roberta didn't do much of anything and continued to drift—after all, she'd done what I asked. Mom, normally the stricter one, was sailing because of her newly discovered sexual preference—she'd become involved with a woman—and now agreed with Dad (who was equally lost in his own supercharged romance). They again decided to give things a chance. Finally, as Roberta's functioning continued to slide, I asked that she go for an evaluation to an expert in kids and drugs. I told the parents that despite everything else going on it *had* to be done, sharing with them my concerns.

From the rigorous evaluation, the secrets she'd been keeping from me and her parents emerged. Roberta was smoking pot several times daily and dating a dealer, and she had recently started doing Ecstasy. She was immediately placed in a program for substance use. Both parents became involved, even as they continued on with their new lives and toward an amicable divorce.

Roberta is an example of why therapists sometimes lose a case when we force the issue of confidentiality. Although we still speak, I no longer see Roberta in treatment. But it was worth it. Roberta gave up substances and the increasingly dangerous life that went with it. She is now going to an excellent public university in town, near her parents.

WHEN KIDS WANT *YOU* TO HANDLE IT

Ideally, you will be able to get a teen to talk to her parents about a dangerous situation. For one reason or another, though she may not be able to speak to Mom and Dad on her own. In such cases, ask whether she will let you handle it.

Natalie, 16½, in a junior year panic, was handling school by getting other kids to do her work. She wanted me to talk to her parents because there was a prohibition in her family against being "weak." Natalie was afraid that by admitting to her terrible performance anxieties, she would be judged harshly. So, she asked me to handle it, because she thought I would convey the information in a way that would minimize her parents' disappointment. Natalie was right to ask me—her parents' reaction was, indeed, harsh; they could not believe *their* daughter was so fragile that she needed extra academic help, help they couldn't afford anyway. It took several meetings for them to understand how tortured Natalie felt, and how debilitating her anxieties were. Finally, a sliding-scale evaluation for medication and learning issues was arranged.

I was seeing Peter, a "good" kid who was not acting out—no drugs, sex or other high-risk behaviors. But Peter had been picked on mercilessly in elementary school. Like numbers of other 21st-century boys who have been bullied, Peter developed a compensatory fantasy world from TV, action comics and video games. Because one of his parents had been diagnosed with a life-threatening illness, and he was under increasing pressure at school, Peter's fantasies were pressing in on him more. After he reacted to a failing grade by taking a paintball gun and splattering his room, I was concerned about whether he was fragmenting. I told Peter I was worried.

PETER: There's nothing wrong with what I'm saying. The paintball stuff was part of my fantasy world.

THERAPIST: Well, it's beginning to sound more real than the way it used to sound. I don't feel comfortable keeping this to myself.

PETER: I don't want you to say anything. I have to say no. I've watched enough TV to realize what my rights are. I'm not in any danger, I'm not going to do anything to myself or anybody else.

THERAPIST: I'm not saying you're going to do something to yourself or anyone else. But, you're wrong. I have a responsibility to say something, even though I know you don't want me to. Try to trust that I'll be able to talk to your parents in a way that isn't going to scare them. I'd like to refer you to a psychiatrist . . . get a second opinion on this. I just don't know what's going on.

PETER: Well, wait till next week when I see you.

THERAPIST: No, that's too long. It takes a lot of time to put together this kind of consultation. Believe me, you're going to feel less concerned when you see how hard it is to find someone who even has openings. I can't tell if you're in danger or not. I don't think you are. But I don't want to take that chance. I like you too much and it's my job.

PETER: I refuse to take medicine.

THERAPIST: It's not my decision whether you take medicine. But I know a psychiatrist who doesn't push medication, and you'll make that decision together with him and your parents."

PETER (*still angry*): All right, all right. You take care of it. But you better tell my parents in a way that doesn't freak them out, because then they'll put even tighter security on me. You got that?

THERAPIST: I appreciate your taking my feelings into account. I'll be extremely careful with them."

I talked to Peter's parents that night. I presented the situation by explaining that he was under increasing pressure at home and school, and his fantasy life was pressing in on him. At first, his mother and father, just like Peter, didn't want to take any of this seriously. I said, "No, for me to continue to work with Peter and to feel comfortable, you really need to go for this consultation. We'll talk about it together. It doesn't mean that he has to take medication. But I must have a second head involved here, someone to compare notes with." The consultation was finally arranged. They all decided against medication, but Peter's allowing me to create a bridge between his anxiety-laden fantasy world and his parents helped him feel better known. We moved beyond this episode, and Peter slowly entered the nitty-gritty world of the second family. *Then* we were in for the dangerous roller-coaster ride that is, by today's standards, normal adolescence—and the real worrying began.

How to Tell Whether Flexible Confidentiality Works

When you do share information with parents, you will quickly know if your openness was helpful or not. In most cases, though not all, if a teen starts acting out more it's an accurate indication that sharing information with parents is wrong. Or, you may share in an incorrect way or betray even small confidences that endanger the relationship. In other words, you receive pretty much immediate feedback about how effectively parents are using information, and about whether you've gone too far.

For example, the more I allowed Fawn's mother into the details of what was going on in her world, the more Fawn would act out—stay out later and push the drinking and hooking-up envelope a lot more. It was uncanny. Even if Fawn had no idea I was talking to her mother, even if her mother mentioned absolutely nothing, Fawn somehow "knew." When another child, Noah, sensed that I was talking to his parents too much (they would drop hints about hearing something regarding his after-school activities), he began to lie to me more often, lie more to teachers about homework, and break more promises to other adults.

On the other hand, after I shared information with the parents of fast-talking Ian about how kids easily twist the truth, Ian respected their newfound "smarts"—they weren't falling for stories about the illegal activities he was up to. And, he clearly felt less guilty about always getting away with everything. When I spoke with Ian's parents, it opened up doors. Ian had been estranged from his father. Since the beginning of treatment, we had many discussions about what I could tell his parents and what I could not. The more I brought Dad in, the more *Ian* talked to Dad about his remarriage after the divorce, jealousy of his baby stepbrother, and why he was unwilling to even visit Dad's new house. For Nicholas, a boy with a depressive disorder, the more I was able to help his mother understand the content of Nick's worries and how to listen better, the more his dark moods were contained with less medication.

*   *   *

Kids' feedback about "flexible-confidentiality" is usually obvious. Lack of any response whatsoever is a disheartening signal. For example, Drew was a boy so deep into a second family of graffiti, grunge concerts, and nihilistic vandalism, my talking to his parents didn't matter one bit. They were so disconnected

from each other's worlds I could have told Mom and Dad anything, and it would have made no difference. Their inability to be
felt as substantial parents, their impotence in the face of adolescent power, was a major reason to focus on parenting strategies—concrete direction many parents *desperately* need, and an
area our field has for too long ignored.

THE PARENT TRAP

Childrearing Advice as Essential to Helping Parents Change Behavior

Ron, why are you writing about parenting? Shouldn't you be devoting your time to more respected areas in the field?
—*A colleague's advice 15 years ago*

Over the past 20 years, I have led hundreds of workshops for mental health professionals around the country. It has been shocking to me how little state-of-the-art or even basic parenting information child professionals are given, although dealing with all-age children demands that we guide parents in crisis—that we be expert on what works and what does not work.

This is a glaring deficit in our training. And, there are several reasons for it. The most obvious is that "parenting" as compared to child development or clinical theory is viewed with intellectual disdain by some clinicians. It suffers from biases our field has held against mothers—too ordinary and too practical. With little research to support it, childrearing techniques were long considered to be in the realm of pop psychology. What's to learn? We were all kids once ourselves, so anyone with a bit of common sense should know what there is to know. Childrearing, *as an integral part of treatment, has clearly not been embraced in our training*. The course offerings of most programs make it apparent how little emphasis is placed on this aspect of the work.

But, frontline child professionals, such as therapists, counselors, caseworkers, school teachers, guidance personnel, and pastoral counselors seem to think differently. Despite less-than-enthusiastic acceptance by mainstream clinical theorists, seminars that integrate clinical issues with concrete parenting techniques have been extremely popular. Tens of thousands of professionals attend my and others' talks on helping parents with basic childrearing matters: how to get kids to listen, how to get adolescents to open up, and how to build self-esteem, among many everyday topics.

These workshops continue to be in such demand for one reason—child professionals are hungry for the content. Counselors simply do not know what to tell parents about creating effective discipline, greater connection, or open communication. In addition, short-lived fads in childrearing (which mirror changing perspectives in clinical practice) have left clinicians almost as confused as parents. Even if our field accepted childrearing advice as part of a helping relationship, we would have to wade through a maze of contradictory advice.

This chapter is structured much like one of my workshops. First, it provides a social/clinical context on different childrearing concerns; second, it describes "what works"—basic parenting techniques that have been proven with kids across most diagnostic categories. The strategies presented create relational traction and behavioral change with the parents of teens—mothers and fathers who desperately look to us for answers during difficult times.

Why You May Be Confused: Five Major Parenting Trends

Parenting advice is informed by evolving theory in psychological thinking. Five major trends have emerged since World War II. Each mirrored the social context and each was greatly affected by clinical developments specific to those times. Each approach made an invaluable contribution, yet also seemed to entirely contradict the approach that preceded it. It is quite a story.

LISTEN TO THE KIDS

Post-World War II psychoanalysis gave rise to the childrearing theories of Haim Ginott (*Between Parent and Child*, 1965) and Thomas Gordon (1970), who founded parent effectiveness training (PET). Almost every major parenting expert who emerged after the '60s was trained by Ginott or his wife, Alice. This psychoanalytically informed view held that children had been squelched and dismissed. They were seen, but not heard. Above all else, kids needed to be listened to. By not listening well, parents failed to validate a child, turning him into the kind of neurotic grown-up that analysts were then treating. The impact of this was profound. PET became a national movement, and its theories spawned thousands of guidance groups across the country, as well as furthering progressive teaching models in early education.

GET TOUGH WITH THE KIDS

During the '70s, partly in reaction to this child-centered focus and partly in reaction to social fragmentation, "tough love" emerged. We are listening entirely too much to children, this philosophy warned, raising kids who "control" parents, instead of the other way around. Tough Love resonated with an apparent truth—the startling increase in acting-out teens. Wild kids were referred to agencies and therapists in droves; disrespect toward authority, adolescent drug use, and teenage pregnancy were epidemic. Consequently, tough love support groups, therapeutic programs, and family therapy put great emphasis on reestablishing parental hierarchy. Mothers and fathers were advised to impose stricter limits on their children, demanding that kids toe the line. My own family systems training in the late '70s was deeply affected by the notion that, for psychic health's sake, we needed to impose order on chaotic family life.

PRAISE THE KIDS

Tough love, too, triggered a national groundswell, yet it also gave way to another perspective: the "self-esteem movement." As hundreds of thousands of adults began to "share and care" in 12-step programs, they talked about previously taboo subjects—family violence, sexual abuse, and addictive and eating disorders, to name just a few. We began to learn about the quiet horrors that went on behind closed doors. Through this national cleansing, Americans discovered how self-esteem is severely damaged by the vicissitudes of dysfunctional family life. At the same time, psychoanalysts Heinz Kohut (*The Analysis of the Self*, 1971) and Alice Miller rocked the psychology, self-help, *and* parenting establishments. Both considered self-esteem a central component of healthy child development. Self-regard must be nurtured in young children or serious pathology will follow. Miller, one of the gurus of the 12-step movement, wrote popularized books (in particular, *Prisoners of Childhood*, 1981) concerning the need to validate each child's uniqueness. Techniques in parenting and education reflected the goal of strengthening a child's self-esteem through acknowledgment, validation, active listening, and praise.

TEACH VALUES TO THE KIDS

Like PET and tough love, the self-esteem movement reached national prominence and, then, spawned a diametrically different perspective. During the '80s, "family values" proponents registered deep dissatisfaction with the self-esteem movement. This notion held that, while children are, indeed, special and unique, what kids really need are old-fashioned virtues: love, honor, courage, loyalty, and honesty. These were among the qualities parents should encourage in children, who were once again thought to be "spoiled rotten" (Fred G. Gosman, 1990). William J. Bennett's *The Book of Virtues* (1993) and Linda and Richard Eyre's *Teaching Your Child Values* (1993) were national best sellers, reflecting public concern that child-centered parenting and progressive education were a threat to the moral fabric of our country's future.

DIAGNOSE AND MEDICATE THE KIDS

Finally, the last trend flew in the face of the moralistic approach that preceded it, and is what I call the "medicalization of childhood." From the early to mid-'90s, advances in understanding body chemistry, temperament, "hard-wiring," and the brain gave rise to a plethora of new diagnoses. Almost every child professional, as well as increasing numbers of educators and parents, are by now familiar with attention-deficit disorder, attention-deficit/hyperactivity disorder, obsessive–compulsive disorder, pervasive developmental disorder, depression, multisensory integration, and, lately, bipolar disorder. Discover the diagnosis and you will know how to treat the child.

Sorting out This Mess

The sheer glut of information, not to mention contradictory views on what parents should provide, created mass confusion! Parents are beside themselves. Professionals, too, are often at a loss about how to incorporate what is valuable—and a lot is very valuable—from each of these childrearing trends. For every problem, there are dozens of different opinions about what ought to be done.

This is where we come in. Child professionals can help integrate the best of these trends into the work we do. Specifically, we must:

♦ Synthesize the five trends of parenting advice.

♦ Offer parents concrete advice regarding what works and what does not, *especially with teens.*

♦ Make suggestions that are practical and clear, so that parents are better able to heal problems on their own.

In the following sections, I outline the most important childrearing techniques we can provide parents of preteens and adolescents.

Privileges Must Be Earned

Privileges are not entitlements; they must be earned. Adolescents *do* need to feel special and listened to. However, this does not translate into the notion, which many parents and kids believe, that specific privileges automatically appear at certain ages.

In 21st-century life, kids expect privileges at developmental milestones. In cities, by late elementary school they clamor to use *public transportation*; in the suburbs, they demand to be dropped off at the mall with friends, *"no adults allowed,"* and picked up hours later. A child turns 13, and he feels entitled to a *curfew*. A 14-year-old believes she should be allowed to hang out with friends *both* nights of the weekend. By 15, *midweek* concerts are considered the norm; at 16 (earlier, in many states), almost all kids expect *to drive*; and, in senior year of high school, a growing ritual across the United States calls for an *unsupervised spring-break*—a week of non-stop debauchery, somewhere, anywhere, without parents.

The notion that "the envelope" automatically opens, that privileges are developmental entitlements rather than something to be earned, is by now a given. Mothers and fathers buy into this idea hook, line, and sinker. Many don't want to be overly restrictive; others feel guilty about long hours at work and away from home. Of course, almost all are pressured by teen litigators: "How can you *not* let me stay out until 1:30! *Every kid* I know stays out *later*. I'm the *only tenth grader* in school who's supposed to be home by *midnight!*" These days, the "everybody's doing it" line actually has more truth to it than several decades ago. Remember, adolescence often looks more like what we used to refer to as "bad behavior"—drinking, experimenting with drugs, smoking, casual hooking up. It's easy to see how parents can be coerced into accepting this mind-set, especially if they are "forbidden" to call other parents and check out reality. Normal adolescence is a dangerous time, one in which a lot of kids end up in treatment, precisely because they are being so ordinary.

Changing a parent's mind-set about "adolescent entitlements" is a critical part of working with just about every teen. We need to get across the idea that privileges must be earned, even though most teens think they are a basic right.

Trust Is a Two-Way Street

Adults often focus on whether or not teens trust them. But, when working with adolescents, the opposite is just as important: Do you trust your teen client? Will he tell the truth to his parents, let them in on some of what's going on, not say whatever he deems necessary, until his parents cave in? These are questions I ask mothers and fathers, who worry so much about whether kids trust them they forget *adult* trust also counts. They forget that trust is a two-way street.

Mike, 15, came to see me after being taken down to police headquarters for vandalism. In fact, that was just the tip of the iceberg. Mike had been involved in a whole range of illicit behaviors, which his parents had no idea about at all. They regularly allowed Mike privileges—unlimited curfew, permission to drive around with other kids, not checking in with them—simply because he was almost 16. In fact, Mike and his pals had been off on extended forays into nearby states where they were involved in a wide range of dangerous mischief.

The arrest jolted Mike's parents into reconsidering their assumptions. They sensed Mike might be abusing privileges, that not everything added up. But they were hesitant to hurt the ostensibly good relationship between them. The combination of Mike's brush with the law and their growing uneasiness made a change of mindset easier: After a month's grounding, Mike needed to *earn* driving privileges back by being home on time, keeping his word about where he was going, and checking in with them exactly when he said he would.

Mike now had to drive on a two-way street regarding trust. Whether his parents trusted Mike became a focus of our work.

Parents Know a Lot More Than They Think

Parents often have the right instincts about when their child is in trouble. Unfortunately, those mothers and fathers whose kids end up in our offices or agencies don't trust themselves. Most adolescents are skilled at planting seeds of doubt. For example, Warren, a glib teenager, was able to run circles around his mom and dad (and most other adults). He was proud of his talent, as were his *parents* about their clever son. Warren said to me, "If my mom and dad were standing in front of a lake, I could absolutely convince them they were standing in front of a mountain."

Between parents and son, there existed a potentially dangerous collusion: Warren's mother and father wanted to provide a more trusting atmosphere than each of them experienced growing up. They *knew* their son was a con artist, but didn't trust their own instincts when an explanation from Warren made little sense. Warren *knew* how to work their denial. He *knew* how badly they wanted to be trusted. He *counted* on their loyalty to him, rather than to their own instincts.

Treatment included getting Warren's mom and dad to take their own reactions seriously when things didn't add up. Over time, yellow flags which had been ignored started to become apparent—Warren's tone of voice, the speed of his delivery, the slightly different stories he doled out to each of them. Warren's suddenly smarter mother and father revoked certain privileges he'd always taken for granted. The boy complained bitterly: "I'm a kid, I'm entitled to do what I want." "No, sorry, you're not," they replied. "Rights no longer automatically come with the territory. They come with handling the responsibility: Respect our curfews, be honest where you're going, tell us at least a couple of names of kids you're actually with, and, then, you'll regain some privileges." Slowly, Warren began to lie less to his mom and dad, who had been his willing dupes. Ignorance at home about life in the second family began to diminish.

Paradoxically, once parents trust their own instincts and "get" that teen privileges must be earned, they often feel more in charge than they did with younger kids. After all, no one is willing to work harder for privileges than a teen who craves being with his second family. And, as I've learned listening to thousands of kids, no one respects intuitive adults more than adolescents.

Consequences Count

Most mental health providers are philosophically and clinically progressive. We think of insight, understanding, cognitive-behavioral exercises, social-emotional protocols, reframing, and so on as key to change. However, childrearing literature and longitudinal studies over the past decade indicate that expectations, not just empathy, are an essential part of the equation.

As I interviewed groups of kids—first, friends of my clients invited into treatment, then 250 kids from nursery school through high school (see my earlier book *Nurturing Good Children Now*, 1999)—I had to accept that consequences actually count. During these sessions I talked to many teens regarding "what works" at home and what gets them to listen to parents. In addition, I spoke with hundreds of principals, teachers, coaches, and other adults who are responsible for the children in our lives. Paraphrasing kids: "All those explanations and teaching lessons aren't enough— we still need consequences." From educators, I heard a similar message: "It's sad to say, but the latest teaching modules about increasing empathy, compassion toward peers, and caution regarding high-risk behaviors—just don't work without some consequences attached." Like me, these professionals were taught to believe otherwise. It is a major change in mind-set for many helping professionals to understand that insight and compassion are not usually sufficient to get ordinary kids to change. It was uncomfortable for me to realize that a critical part of the work must be teaching parents how to *effectively create consequences*.

Most often, by the time a teen has entered therapy, mothers and fathers have absolutely no idea about what to do. They have tried reason, discussion, and threats. They have already taken away everything they can. Nothing seems to work. Other, more lenient parents think consequences are appropriate for younger children, but not for teens—who must learn about life from their own experiences. At the same time, adolescents are often great poker players—they'll call an adult's bluff, saying in so many words, "Anything you do won't have an effect on me. I'm going to live my life the way I want to!" For harried, confused parents this attitude is effective enough to turn determined consequences into unenforceable threats.

Given the many forces that can undermine adult authority, here is how to help parents create consequences that matter to teens.

Teens Give Parents All the Leverage They Need

About a dozen years ago, I realized that parents of teens actually have much more leverage than they realize. Why? *Adolescent life is always about the next big thing on the horizon, the next "If I don't go I'll die" event*—the prom, the biggest party, the most major rock concert ever! E-mails fly, phones ring, text messages and beepers digitally connect. Plans are secretly hatched, rehatched, and hatched once again. The endless possibilities of adolescence are what scares parents half to death. But kids' tunnel vision also provides powerful leverage for mothers and fathers.

Counseling parents to use "the next big event" as a consequence puts them in a far more effective position. A big event doesn't have to be what we as adults might consider huge, such as the junior prom. It can be the basketball game on Saturday, a trip to the mall, or even an afternoon "chilling" with friends. When a parent finds the courage to say, "You can't go, because you didn't stick to our agreement last week about your curfew," that parent discovers hidden power in what so often feels like an out-of-whack equation.

Noreen, 14, had many psychological issues: mercurial moods, ruminative episodes, and a hot-and-cold attitude about school. Her issues, however, did not prevent Noreen from wanting to go out with friends two or three times a week, to drink and smoke dope, or to stay out way past curfew. Noreen's mother, Robin, was overwhelmed. Noreen usually announced her plans at the last possible minute—"I'm going to Jen's house with a few other kids! OK?" Robin felt she had little control over her comings and goings. If Mom even mildly protested about these 11th-hour requests Noreen objected. Robin became crazed, screaming unenforceable threats and insults she regretted the moment they left her lips. Noreen, in turn, became wild too, adamantly defending her right to go out and do whatever she wanted. In our meetings alone, Robin reexamined the "entitlement rationale," how furious it made her, and began considering whether to trust her own instincts when things didn't add up. After a while, Mom saw that greater leverage with Noreen existed right in front of her face. Finally, she calmly said, "Noreen, you didn't come back at the time we agreed on last week. In fact, when you came in, you seemed a little out of it. So, you won't be able to go out this weekend."

The diatribes and counterthreats began, but Robin stuck to the consequence—which required several between-session calls to me. Noreen refused to talk and spent even more time online with friends, bitching about her "maniacal" mother. In meetings with Noreen, I asked how she felt, but also empathized with her mother's need to take a stand: "You're good—you've got your mother plenty worried." "Look, I know she's not easy to live with when she's so upset." "The more you work with her, the more you'll get in return." Noreen glared, but she didn't bolt. As Robin held firm, Noreen coincidentally opened up a little about matters heretofore reserved only for friends and me—a hidden tattoo, experimenting with smoking up, constantly changing alliances with girlfriends. This was more a negotiating ploy than real candor, but it was a beginning. Robin began to open her eyes to her own power and the hidden realities of second-family life. Noreen calmed down just enough to start her long journey towards greater self-regulation.

CONSEQUENCES MUST BE SPECIFIC

Noreen and Robin's situation is far from unique. Parents are often vaguely aware of the next big event on the horizon; they've heard their child talking about it to friends or, if they pay attention, clues are left here and there. So, if it's necessary to impose a consequence, it ought to be specifically related to the particular happening: "I'm sorry, you can't go to the Modest Mouse concert this Saturday. You didn't keep your word when you went to that "chilling" party last weekend. You told us the party would be small and your friend's parents would be there. Instead 300 kids showed up and there were no adults at all. There's another concert coming up in a month. You'll be able to go to that if you keep your word about curfews between now and then."

The point is, vague consequences are usually ineffective. Non-specific, frustration-fueled consequences are hard to enforce and tend to backfire, usually making life harder on a parent. Teens see unenforceable threats as a red flag, announcing: "Don't take me seriously!"

There's a bonus to specific consequences: Parents learn more about what is really going on behind the wall of silence. Very often, a typically closed-mouth adolescent will start talking, while trying to renegotiate rights. For example, 15-year-old Hannah, desperate to get to a friend's 16th-birthday party, suddenly admitted that kids did, indeed, drink "a little" at these parties, and that she herself had tried a beer once or twice. But, if allowed to go, she would "absolutely not drink a drop that weekend." This admission was, of course, a pose. Hannah had absolutely no intention to give up drinking, a gray-zone behavior contributing to her falling grades and morose mood. Hannah was spilling the beans to get what she wanted. With my encouragement, the consequence stuck. In the process, I helped Mom open her eyes to the reality of the hard partying that had been hinted at during Hannah's desperate negotiation over the consequences.

The Parent Realist

Adolescents are contemptuous of unrealistic limits, mindlessly imposed by adults—parents, teachers, and therapists. Teens correctly recognize a false threat as the effort of a parent who doesn't know his or her inability to control what happens behind the wall of silence. Being unrealistic with an adolescent is corrosive; it eats away at connection. This is why kids often seem closer to parents *after* a realistic limit has been enforced. I have heard stories about thousands of kids who will snuggle, sit on a lap, or start opening up—immediately following a stormy, limit-setting confrontation. Being "the parent realist," doesn't only change behavior by establishing appropriate hierarchy, it also creates genuine connection.

To be realistic, all limits about consequences should contain the following three components:

HELP PARENTS TO BE CLEAR
ABOUT THEIR EXPECTATIONS

Childrearing research and longitudinal studies demonstrate that clarity counts for a lot. Most kids don't even register expectations if delivered angrily or ambiguously. That means saying, "You can go to the dance, but I don't want you to drink. I don't believe it's safe." "I'd like you home by 5:30; that's 5:30 P.M. A few minutes later and we have a problem." "Call me by midnight to tell me where you are. I will be near the phone. Please call on time."

HELP PARENTS ADMIT THEIR RELATIVE IMPOTENCE

Parental control is severely limited in the 21st century. It is more powerful to admit one's impotence and to focus on our own limits than to focus exclusively on limits for kids. Teens suddenly pay attention when I say, "No adult will be there to monitor; it's ultimately *your* choice." The same goes for parents. *Accepting their own limits paradoxically strengthens the limits they set for teens.*

That means admitting in no uncertain terms: "I can't stop you . . . ," "I'm not going to be there to supervise you . . . ," "I realize it's ultimately going to be your choice, not mine." Acknowledging limits breaks through to teens and creates relational traction because it is true; there *is* nothing a parent can do to stop a child from drinking at the dance, smoking up afterward, driving with unlicensed drivers, signing into chat rooms, having sex, or whatever else may come his or her way. The earlier parents recognize their own limits, the less it feels like an admission of failure. It's just the way it is.

HELP PARENTS SAY,
". . . BUT THERE WILL BE CONSEQUENCES"

As adolescents choose to engage in specific behaviors in the moment, they must know also that consequences will follow if parents' requests are ignored. Kids need to hear what will happen (or that something as-yet undecided will happen) *if* they go against parents' expectations.

The third part of the message, then, is "I won't be there, but if I sense or find out you were smoking pot, there will be a consequence. I don't know what it will be yet, but something will happen."

"I can't always be driving with you. But if you get just one speeding ticket, it becomes *our* license for the next six months."

Even complex issues, such as eating disorders, require that adults become more realistic in their approach. One anorexic teen I worked with made improvements when the girl's mother and physician began saying: "You need to eat a little more. We now know we can't make you. We can't be with you at lunchtime in school. We can't be there before the weigh-in, to see if you put change in your pockets or drink a lot of water. We're not around at other people's houses. It's up to you. *But, the weight we agreed on must be maintained. If you drop below that weight you're going to the hospital.*" The combination of a clear expectation, recognition of adult limits, and a consequence were just enough to keep this girl out of the hospital, giving her time to overcome her bout with anorexia.

Beyond "Eyes Wide Shut": Help Parents See the Small Stuff

Posttragedy investigations almost always reveal a simple truth: Parents and other adults saw signs of trouble, but they let them go. The small details mattered; they were there to be seen, but few took them seriously or knew what to do.

As child professionals, we have been trained to report the larger realities. For example, as discussed in the chapter on confidentiality, an issue needs to be shared if and when it poses a danger. Similarly, parents are advised to watch out for *red-flag signals*: loss of appetite, change in sleeping and eating patterns, plummeting school grades.

By that time, it is often too late. We needn't wait for these dramatic signals. The research shows that details about what is happening behind the wall of silence are usually on display right in front of parents. This is one of the ironies of working with adolescents. They are so "out there," they can't help but tip their hands. After all, they are still teenagers. Drama, sloppiness, disorganization, self-absorption, memory lapses, frenetic schedules—all create a road map of clues. Kids count on sightless adults not to notice, to keep our "eyes wide shut."

HELP PARENTS PAY ATTENTION TO THE SMALL DETAILS— AND ACT ON THEM

How small? A teen has a 12 A.M. curfew and arrives home 20 minutes late; an adolescent client with a 4 P.M. appointment ambles in to your session 15 minutes past the appointment time. In these situations, it is often true that during those few minutes between promptness and lateness, "something happened." Lateness is not accidental; there is a reason for it. And it behooves parents and counselors to pay attention.

A mother told me that once she began "sweating small stuff," she noticed that whenever her 16-year-old daughter came home from a night out she was chewing gum. This small detail, combined with her daughter's immediate disappearance into her room without a goodnight kiss, helped Mom realize that she might be smoking. In fact, Mom was belatedly correct; it had been going on for almost a year "without notice."

Another parent told me that she suddenly picked up on the way her child held a bottle of soda around the dinner table. Upon reflection, the girl seemed to be posing, unconsciously mirroring the way kids hold bottles of beer when they drink. For months, this teen had been cluing her mother in to the fact that she was regularly involved with the world of clubbing at illegal after-hours bars and with weekend cocaine use.

A boy's taste in music changed abruptly. Instead of the classic-rock his father introduced him to, he started to like punk and anarchist bands. Dad didn't notice. He still didn't register the cynicism his son spouted about all institutions, including school, chalking it up to ornery adolescence. Only later, when he began cutting classes (Dad was finally notified by the school after over 50 classes had been cut—a not uncommon experience; overburdened schools also only have the time to spot red flags, not these yellow ones). Finally, Dad *had* to notice when his son began lifting entire term papers off the Internet. By the time he connected all the dots, real trouble had, in fact, been going on for a long time.

Parents know teens better than they realize. Eyes are wide shut because they don't *want* to pay attention. What they sense is just too scary or disappointing to think about, let alone to act on. Parents need to be encouraged to pay attention, because the details matter. The earlier kids are seen clearly, the less they lie and the less they drift out to the true dangers of the second family.

Solution Seeking Works

As Myrna Shure's research shows when parents and children are able to find solutions together, they move more easily through the rocky shoals of ordinary life (Raising a Thinking Child, 1994).

We see this in our counseling rooms every day. An adolescent presents for treatment, and there's usually little ability of parent and teen to come up with solutions jointly. Indeed, much observational research in family therapy shows that the inability to make decisions is a key indicator of individual or systemic pathology—with rage and anxiety often taking over. This means we must help parents develop skills to concretely discuss solutions about dealing with a clique at school or approaching a tough teacher or a bossy queen bee. Unfortunately, therapists (like academic tutors) don't always share these skills with parents, even though mothers and fathers live with the child 99% of the time.

We can teach collaborative solution seeking in two major ways: *First, by sharing with parents the learning channels we discover about their kids in individual meetings.* For example, since debate worked wonders with Collette, I practiced with her dad the art of arguing without becoming abrasive. With a 12-year-old who refused "linear" directives, I showed her straight-shooting mom how to create the "limited-choice" scenario her daughter responded to: "You can either get dressed first or comb your hair out later—you choose." I helped anxious Maria's mother and father see that solutions to peer dilemmas work best if they are realistic ("This may not help") rather than falsely reassuring ("I'm sure your argument with Carlos will disappear").

Second, teens often balk at parental solutions, because we haven't asked how we can be helpful—or what they might need from us. Therefore, I "tutor" parents about how to ask kids to let us help them.

Rules of Engagement:
Active Problem Solving with Teens

♦ Always approach during a calm moment.

♦ Approach with no siblings around.

♦ Say clearly, "I don't know the answer to this, so maybe you can help I me."

♦ Acknowledge the child's feeling: "I can see how _____ you feel!"

♦ Check it out: "Is that right?"

♦ "How do you think we can handle it differently?"

♦ If the child has no ideas, say, "I've been thinking—here are a couple of solutions I've come up with—what do you think?"

♦ If no success, try again later, while engaged together in a calm activity.

For example, Jason's parents could not get their son up in the morning. Whatever they did, nothing would rouse him. So, Jason arrived late at school every day, one semester accumulating almost

70 late notices. He started cutting even more classes, teachers were furious, and Jason was in danger of being left back. Collaborative efforts to find solutions seemed almost as important as the solution itself—which ended up being quite a surprise.

Jason's parents followed the guidelines in the Rules of Engagement box. We were all surprised by the result. Since Jason became furious at whoever tried to wake him, when asked what *he* thought might work (the first time he'd ever been asked), Jason suggested that the family dog could get him moving. "How could I get mad at my puppy in the morning?" Jason was right. His attendance record improved just enough to pass—only 20 recorded latenesses. Though this improvement was pretty radical, it was not as revolutionary as the idea that a heretofore insolent adolescent might be able to come up with his own creative solution.

Help Parents Listen Better

It is a myth that teens do not open up to parents. However, it is *not* a myth that parents are often poor listeners. John Gottman's research focusing on communication between family members documents what clinicians have sensed for some time: Adults must significantly improve their listening skills. Compared to the second family, parents are at best neutral, at worst maddening, listeners. I share this "fact of family life" with every group of parents I address. The bottom line? Most mothers and fathers recognize how often they sabotage good listening—anger, fear, worry, impatience, the memory of our own experience as adolescents—all get in the way. They admit to confusion over contradictory advice about listening: Should I drop everything? Will my emotions crowd out my kid? If I disagree, will my child never talk to me again? If I don't disagree, am I being a doormat? Am I overreacting? Of course, parents also complain about how kids open up at the most difficult moments: at bedtime, in the middle of heated negotiations over privileges, when they deeply disappoint parents, or when they simmer with rage and scream searing truths about us.

Despite poor listening skills, adult confusion, and the awful timing of adolescents, there are now consistent guidelines to help parents keep the lines of communication open.

DON'T POUNCE

Twelve-year-old Brian put it this way: "My mom is so into 'communication,' if I just *open* my mouth, she'll *pounce* on me to have a *talk*. It makes me feel like *puking*, and I immediately want to get away."

Now that's a pretty pungent reaction, so I asked Brian why he felt so strongly: "It begins to feel like talking is *more important to her* than it is to me."

Communication-starved parents jump on a child the second he wants to talk. Many mothers and fathers could be in the middle of performing a brain operation, but—"My teenager wants to talk? I'll stop what I'm doing. If I blow this opportunity, he'll never speak to me again." Parents need to learn that opportunities arise continuously—especially so with teens—who always want the next big thing.

DON'T NECESSARILY "NAME A CHILD'S FEELINGS"

Once a conversation begins, help parents avoid falling into the "therapist dance": to "validate" a child's experience. That reflective technique, long a staple of childrearing advice, has merits. But it should be reserved for a child's more troubled moments, not for ordinary closed-mouthed teens. Kids who are in a panic need this quasi-therapeutic technique. But, saying too often "You must be feeling angry" or "You must feel sad" gets old real soon. For example, 12-year-old Bobbie tells Mom that a friend openly criticized him in front of the other kids at school. If mom responds by saying yet again "Oh, that must have made you feel very angry," there's a good chance that Bobbie will answer, "Uh-huh," and move off into another room. Distance, rather than a relational connection, has been unwittingly created.

ASK ACTION-ORIENTED QUESTIONS

What happened then? What did you do next? She said that? How did it end? All questions aim at the action—not the feelings—and help a child tell his or her "story." You must have faith that a child's emotions are going to emerge from adult *interest* in the story line that unfolds. It has been said that "love is focused interest." Focusing on action lets the story, and with it feelings, beliefs, and interpretations, come out. Teens, especially, need to develop "emotional literacy," the ability to describe experience through words, not acting out. So action-questions help. Encourage angry, impatient parents not to editorialize, analyze, or "fix" before the plot becomes clear. Teens are natural dramatists. They respond to anyone who is initially interested in the story line, not the *feelings* first. They experience traction with an interested listener.

DON'T ASK "WHY?"

This is a big temptation for outraged, disappointed parents. When you get right down to it, even adults who have been trying to figure themselves out for decades do not really know why we do a lot of the things we do! Most kids don't have a clue either. One day, while sorting socks, Daphne told her mother that a group of kids made fun of her at dancing class. Mom was tempted to stop their parallel conversation, sit her daughter down, and ask, "Well, *why* didn't you walk away or tell the teacher?" That would have dead-ended the discussion. Instead, as I had suggested, Mom went on with sock sorting, asked action-oriented questions, and stayed focused on *what actually happened.* Rather than closing down, her daughter couldn't stop from describing the details, in the process revealing more and more of her feelings and interpersonal dilemmas.

HELP PARENTS RESPOND

This is crucial to developing relational traction. If you look at several of the post-World War II models of childrearing, a parent is supposed to be laid back, so as not to overpower. But, in fact, kids don't feel "held" until we *respond* to them. This is a totally opposite notion than the idea of giving kids "space" to have their feelings.

When Daphne finished relating her story, Mom, in a most untherapeutic fashion, expressed her honest reaction: "That's *awful!* I *can't stand* those girls for picking on you." As soon as Daphne was responded to with genuine emotion, she felt heard. Later that evening, Mom and Daphne sat down to figure out how to handle the problem.

Prepare Parents for Conflict Discussions

Teen timing is, indeed, awful for parents—kids usually open up in the midst of conflict. Preparing mothers and fathers for this can turn high conflict into moments that may loosen stuck interactions. Remind parents that teens talk at the following times:

♦ *When they scare parents.* I learned this lesson years ago from Audrey, whose son, Billy, had been secretly experimenting with hallucinogens, marijuana, and hashish. Audrey was a progressive parent; she had told Billy it was all right to experiment with pot, and normal to occasionally drink. But she emphatically told him to stay away from LSD—anything but acid. It was too frightening; it could destroy him psychically. Of course, LSD was exactly what Billy tried. He returned home in a panic, which was absolutely terrifying to his mother, who had seen too many of her '60s friends go through terrible "trips," never to return. Audrey told me: "No matter how scared I was, I knew I had to listen. I had to push back all my fears, forget about the fact that I repeatedly warned him to stay away from this stuff. I had to swallow hard and hear what he was saying." Years later, Billy confided to me that this moment—when his mother held back her own fear and just listened—was a turning point in their relationship. It was when he began to *get* that his mom truly meant well for him. Billy moved beyond that early-adolescent "she's against me" mind-set, realizing that Audry was not just another adult out to control him.

♦ *When they disappoint parents the most*. Kids tend to open up when they have gone precisely against values parents have tried to instill in them. Often, when adults are the most disappointed in kids, the potential for real communication also exists.

Maureen had moved to a ritzy new neighborhood. She had told her children in her usual no-nonsense, authoritative way, "The last thing I want in this fancy neighborhood is to be publicly humiliated." *The next day* cops pulled up in her driveway! The boys had gotten caught trespassing on someone else's property—a minor infraction, but mom was livid. In reaction to her rage and disappointment, Adam and Nick finally admitted that they were angry, too, at having been uprooted so many times to follow Dad in his jobs. They had never talked about this before—it only came out when they got mom to be terribly disappointed in their behavior.

That is typical of adolescents, but as seven-year-old Bart's story demonstrates, it can happen with younger kids, too. Bart was caught stealing a toy car from another child's house. His parents were hurt and disappointed; they regarded honesty as a very important quality. But, out of the angry confrontation that followed, Bart—a very bright, articulate child who kept his feelings to himself—started talking about how jealous he had always been of his younger brother. His sibling had the sunny looks and disposition that made everybody take notice. The clash and their genuine response seemed to jar his feelings loose.

♦ *When they are embroiled with parents in negotiations*. Thirteen-year-old Anna wanted to go to a party. But her mother thought it was too late to be out. They first got into angry words, which turned into a shouting match and then an all-out war. They screamed at one another; Anna threatened to run away. Finally, Anna's mother actually lay down in front of the door, blocking her exit.

It was a horrible scene, but after it was all over, they sat on the couch together. In tears, Anna came out with what really had been bothering her: Having a learning disability, she constantly struggled to fit into the high-pressure school she attended. Unbeknownst to her mother, the other kids in school had been making fun of Anna for being "stupid." The party was a way of trying to belong. It might have been months before Anna admitted this, or she could have raised a "red flag" by getting into more serious trouble. But the mother–daughter fight around negotiating became a catalyst that helped them get to what was really on Anna's mind.

Teach Parents How to Give Advice

The idea that parental advice is toxic to teens (much like therapeutic advice; see Chapter 5) is another childrearing myth. In fact, adolescent honesty, coming as it does in the midst of crisis, feels incomplete to many teenagers *without* some attempt at adult guidance. It is not easy to read these moments as requests for advice. The "Tell me what you think I should do" subtext is dwarfed by the screaming teen anthem "Leave me alone; get out of my life!" But "Tell me what you think" is just as real. Unfortunately, if parents and other adults are poor at listening, we are even more inept in the guidance department.

How do you help parents get through to kids who act so independent and "adolescent" from the time they've begun grade school? *The answer is in the packaging.* Parents need to package advice in ways modern kids can absorb.

BE BRIEF

Children have been brought up on special effects, remote controls, lightning-fast editing, and MTV. Like it or not, kids often have an attention span based on sound bites and nanoseconds. Parents (and therapists) have, perhaps, three or four sentences to make the point before a teen's mind begins to wander. If a parent repeats herself or takes too long, she will lose the window of opportunity, and perhaps her son's consciousness. Not a word will be heard, and service will be cut off, with nothing more than a dial tone.

So, teach parents the signs that they are talking too long: A teen's got that empty expression; her eyes have rolled up to the ceiling. She may appear to be paying attention, but if you observe closely, she is actually studying your chin or nose or forehead. Therefore, advice need not be repeated more than one extra time, or one decibel louder to get through. Helping parents respect these signals, so obvious in hindsight, is a major accomplishment.

KEEP 'EM WANTING MORE

Parents ought not linger or treat each conversation as if it will be the last opportunity to talk. Tell *mothers and fathers* to end conversations; encourage *parents* to leave kids first. As the old show business expression goes, "Keep 'em begging for more." Remember what one teen said earlier: "Communication shouldn't seem more important to a parent than it does to a child."

This is easier said than done. Parents who have been relentlessly ignored by their teens want to hold on to the moment. It may have been the first good exchange in months; it begs to be savored, so they try to make the conversation last just a little too long. Predictably a teen has already moved away—once more ensconced behind the wall of silence. Therefore, when a talk is over, let it be over. As kids say—"It's old!" Repetition doesn't make for relational traction.

TRY NOT TO BRING UP THE CONVERSATION AGAIN

Certain postconversation questions are deadly: "What did you feel about what I said?" or "Have you been thinking about what we discussed?" or "Wasn't that conversation we had yesterday great?" A parent trying to make sure he got through is looking for trouble and will probably feel hurt when a child looks vacant and says, "What are you talking about?" Half the time she won't remember or will say that to a parent, anyway. Children live in the present and the future. They don't relish "good communication." They don't say, "Thank you." They just grow from it. Ironically, a sign that the conversation worked is that life simply goes on. So should parents.

TRY NOT TO EXPECT GREATER CLOSENESS

Nothing is logical or linear in family life, especially with teens. Close moments do not lead to harmony. Therefore you should prepare parents for this. The same child who was crying on dad's shoulder two hours ago could be locked in mortal combat with him two hours later over a new video game or favoring a younger brother.

It is unwise to fool parents or yourself as a professional into thinking that one conversation—*the* conversation—will make a big difference in cementing relationships. The accumulation of moments in the midst of tension, control struggles, weekend crises, and endless wrangling over privileges strengthens the connection between parent and child. It is a relatively slow process, one I measure in "seasons" (e.g., "Let's see how we all get through this spring"), rather than in sessions.

"I CAN'T MAKE YOU TALK—BUT I CAN WORK ON MYSELF"

As I described earlier, helping professionals need to encourage parents to accept their *own* limits with adolescents. This includes the area of communication: "I can't make *you* talk. I have to work on listening better *myself* . . . ," "I won't be perfect, but *I'll keep trying* not to interrupt or lecture . . . ," "I want you to tell me as much as you can about your life—*I'll figure out* how to deal with it, because I love you."

Statements of intention may be impossible for most resentful or pressured parents to initially consider. Each side is waiting for the other to blink, believing themselves to be right. But, such statements are a powerful message and wonderful modeling that is not lost on kids. Only the most distant teen in the darkest corners of second-family life—chronic drug or alcohol abuse, illegal behavior, or kids with undiagnosed clinical syndromes (bipolar and dual diagnoses, anxiety and depressive disorders) don't secretly welcome this statement. Though they won't register a parent's statement of intention, teens don't forget. The next explosion or disappointment will be accompanied by close scrutiny to see whether a parent can deliver the goods—less hysteria, better listening, more realistic advice.

This statement was not lost on 16-year-old Auriana, who refused to listen to *anything*. After her mom, Madeline, announced her intention to work on *herself,* Madeline interrupted just a little less and spoke with a slightly softer tone of voice. Yes, Mom occasionally relapsed into her managerial style, but each time she avoided the old "yelling dance" with Auriana, this impossible teen became calmer and less combative. It was shocking, even to me, to see what a difference Madeline's "trying" made. Auriana had been on the way to school failure and had been staying at unknown friends' houses for days at a time, but her fast-track life began to slow down just a bit. Within a few months Mother realized they were spending more time watching TV, hanging out, and even casually discussing Auriana's real-life dramas, without much fanfare.

Honor Thy Father and Mother—and Thyself

Physical or verbal abuse by parents is always to be taken seriously. But 21st-century kids are chronically abusive to parents and it hardly registers—"they're just being adolescents." Abuse may be blatantly physical or it may be subtle: rarely speaking, never hearing, demanding attention in harsh terms, being haughty and viciously sarcastic to parents and younger siblings.

Teen verbal barbs are often intended to wound. Fourteen-year-old Holly made fun of the way her overweight mother dressed. Mark, 13, screamed at his mother, "You're such a bitch, no wonder Daddy died, you'll never get another man." Fourteen-year-old Jocelyn said to her mom, "Now, I see why Dad left you for another woman." An adolescent said to his father, "You're a total wimp, of course Mom became a lesbian." Another to his parents: "You fucked me up so much, now you have to make it up to me." Another: "You're so stupid, that's why you don't have any friends— just like I don't."

A purple haze of teenage abuse settles on the house and goes unaddressed or is met with equally intense parental rage. This is another misconception that breeds distance, wider swings into the far reaches of the second family and greater parental ineffectiveness. Verbal abuse of parents pushes kids away. Contempt about being able to say whatever comes to mind reduces the worth of the adults at home. *Life with teens does not have to be this way, nor should it be.* Parents need to change their pop psychology mind-set that it's normal for teens—and themselves—to go for the emotional jugular; they must be guided to stop this "dance of anger" (as Harriet Lerner called it, in marriage and relationship life) with some degree of conviction that it's not acceptable.

Why is it so hard to stop? Parents put up with abuse for many reasons: They feel remorse over their own toxic outbursts; conversely they believe it is important for a child to get emotions off his chest or things will fester and lead to neuroses. Many feel it is unavoidable, in the realm of raging hormones and, therefore, cannot be controlled. Some parents feel terrible guilt about not being around enough or about childrearing errors. Unfortunately, parents all make mistakes with kids, not just small mistakes, but ones with consequences that last years. *When it comes to raising kids, there are as many reasons to feel guilty as there are stars in the sky.*

So, parents feel they deserve some abuse *and* they fear that squelching expressiveness is going to make an adolescent nastier. Just the opposite is true. As kids tell me privately and in group interviews, when they're allowed to say whatever comes to mind, they simply fall apart. "No rules leads to chaos," said one articulate fifth grader. A teenage girl said to me, "I watched my friend Christie snap at her mother yesterday and all of a sudden I saw how mean I am to my mother. I hate Mom for allowing it, and I hate myself for doing it."

For their own good, then, here's how to help kids reign themselves in.

NAME IT

Our kids grow up in a disrespectful culture. "Dissing" is the currency of popularity. They bring home rough-and-tumble schoolyard chatter, e-mail insults, talk-radio rants and demeaning put-downs—*with-*

out even recognizing it! Until a parent or teacher names the behavior, kids (and parents) don't always realize exactly what was out of line.

- ♦ Felicia's mom needed to be reminded that "skank" was not acceptable as a description of her, even if Felicia was angry and felt compelled to express herself.

- ♦ Frederick's dad needed to hear that calling him a "wuss" in front of friends was completely out of line and would not bolster his son's masculinity.

- ♦ Alvin's mother had to be reminded that insults were not a normal part of negotiating privileges, even if her son desperately wanted to go to the concert.

Parents must then say the obvious: "Talking to me that way is disrespectful. I don't like it. And it hurts." Kids of all ages need to hear this because they don't always recognize the impact of their words. A fish is the last to see that it swims in the ocean.

STEP OUT OF THE DANCE

Jeremiah and his mother, Betty, were locked in a vicious battle. Jeremiah assaulted her with a verbal arsenal that could well have been on one of those uncensored talk-show videos, calling mom "a bitch" and blaming her for his father's death—which led to Betty's equally wild recriminations toward Jeremiah. This toxic dance continued for years and was considered normal by both. Jeremiah's mother needed to stop her own reflexive response, name his behavior, and immediately discontinue *any* further conversation. She first attempted to walk away from him, but Jeremiah followed her around the house. With my encouragement, Betty learned to catch her own runaway reactions and disconnect—smile, put on earphones, call a friend, or take a short bath behind a locked door. Even this change was difficult because, to Betty, walking away was equated with total abandonment. After several meetings with me, she finally got it right. Almost immediately, Jeremiah toned down his act and a wary truce set in. Real conversation could now begin.

When Holly launched sarcastic diatribes about her mother's style and appearance, Rhea needed to say: "You can keep criticizing me this way (remembering the limits of her power), but then I don't feel like being nice to you." The tables were turned—Rhea stopped talking to her daughter for the night (easy, since she was so furious herself) and actually "forgot" to make Holly's favorite dessert. Not exactly high-tech, but a powerful message that Holly's contempt would not encourage her mother's ineffective rage or her generosity, either.

Helping Mom to step out of the abusive dance was a revolutionary moment in their lives. It was a turning point toward the pair treating each other more kindly. It allowed the first family at home to develop some "gravitas." Holly coincidentally began staying home a little more often and did not so desperately try to hang out with the popular, mean girls.

Toning Down Parents' Anger

Teach parents this stepwise method to get on top of their reflexive rage:

- Identify early warning signals of danger—there's almost always a physiological tip-off: tight chest, tense jaw, stomach churning, etc.
- Say to oneself—"I'm about to lose it."
- Announce to child—"I need to calm *myself* down."
- Walk away—engage in self-soothing behavior, use trial and error approach to discover what calms.
- If child follows, say, "I can't talk now. The answer is automatically 'no' if you don't leave me alone."
- Explain later, when calmer, that you're working on yourself—controlling your own angry responses.
- Keep trying—eventually your body and teen will get the message.

Note: If this sequence makes no dent, it is time for the parent to consult with a counselor who specializes in anger management.

IMPOSE CONSEQUENCES, CONSISTENT OR OTHERWISE

Holly's mom imposed a natural consequence—"You're not nice to me, I won't go out of my way for you." But often verbal abuse requires a consequence that has impact, though it may not "fit the crime." *A need to be consistent is another myth that ties parents into ineffective knots.* Abuse can be curtailed by removing coveted privileges that have absolutely no connection with the event itself—cutting off TV, taking back car keys, disconnecting e-mail, suspending allowance for weekend activities, among many others. If enforceable, and tied to a parent's sense of being treated badly, illogical consequences are viewed by teens as an entirely logical sign of strength. Interestingly, it was only after 16-year-old Kaleb's parents stopped his trash-talk toward them, that he began to invite his friends over to the house. As long as Mom and Dad felt entitled to be treated well, Kaleb kept bringing kids over to meet them. The moment they slipped, Kaleb started hanging out at other people's homes.

This three-step plan to cut down teen abuse usually works immediately:

1. Name the objectionable behavior.

2. Remove oneself.

3. Impose an enforceable consequence.

When this sequence doesn't work, it's almost a sure sign of unaddressed parental dynamics (for example, a multigenerational history of abuse), an undiagnosed disorder in parent or child (such as anxiety or impulsive-type ADD), or an untreated addiction. An evaluation for these diagnostic concerns is indicated.

Help Parents Praise Kids Effectively

The research on motivation and self-esteem is becoming increasingly clear. Martin E. P. Seligman's *The Optimistic Child* (1995) and Edward L. Deci's *Why We Do What We Do* (1995), discuss the impact of "the self-esteem movement" that began in the '70s. *It is shocking to learn that the more automatic, effusive and hyperbolic the praise, the less kids want to do and the less good they feel about themselves.* Indeed, adult praise has reached epidemic proportions. Children, starting at very young ages become inured to it, dependent on it, and used to instant gratification. Glowing words that endlessly flow from adults make little difference. Adolescents, being acutely conscious of phoniness, resent hollow kudos. They know the real score and it makes them distrust us even more. The key aspect of praise that matters most to teens involves their attempts at self-regulation, as described in the following section.

RECOGNIZE EFFORTS TO SELF-REGULATE

Researchers who focus on temperament tell parents to praise when a child *tries* to contain his hard-wired impulses: bossiness, tenacity, shyness, activity level, pessimism, sensitivity, and so on. With teens, whose lifelong temperamental issues are exponentially inflamed, it is especially important to praise this kind of effort. Even minor attempts to rein themselves in are terribly difficult for adolescents and are behaviors most deserving of praise.

For example, when Alexis arrived home exactly on time Saturday evening, (her first punctual appearance ever), I asked her mother, Lois, later: "Did you say anything to Alexis about it? I imagine it was tough for Alexis to peel herself away. From what I hear, a lot was going on with her friends, and *she always has a hard time not being accommodating.*" Alexis' mom said, "Well, actually I didn't. I was so relieved, I just gave her a kiss." I suggested to Lois: "Sometime in the next day or two, tell Alexis, 'It really made me feel good that you stuck by our agreement on the curfew. I guess it was probably hard for you.'" Lois was stunned at how much Alexis softened after this acknowledgment.

Warren, our silver-tongued con man, spoke back to his hard-driving coach in his typical scathing way. Warren was briefly suspended from the team. Sometime later—in the middle of a basketball game that his dad, Joseph, was attending—the coach rode Warren hard. This time Warren was able to contain himself from reacting sarcastically. Warren's dad saw his son's struggle to hold back, and was extremely pleased. I asked Joseph if he had acknowledged his boy's effort to sit on his lifelong, almost reflexive sassing of adults. Dad realized that he had not, and gave a small nod toward Warren later that evening. It meant a lot to his son and, not coincidentally (he mentioned dad's acknowledgment to me in our meeting), Warren was never rude to his coach again.

Nan, a 12-year-old with moderate attentional issues was finally able to study half an hour straight without procrastinating or putting up an explosive argument. I asked her parents, "What did you say about that?" Their reply: "Well, nothing. We just sort of

---

Resilient Self-Esteem for 21st-Century Kids

- Avoid hyperbole—from three and up, kids know better.
- Avoid "constructive" criticism—teens rarely hear the positive message.
- Praise effort, not product—research shows kids are very aware when they've tried hard or haven't.
- Character generalizations wound—you're "no-good," "lazy," "mean," and the like; they hurt and may become self-fulfilling prophesies.
- Praise indirectly—many kids respond better to nonintimate praise: e-mails, notes, overheard conversations.
- "I'm proud of you" doesn't cut it for most teens. . . . It feels like it's about us, not them.
- Honest, gently delivered feedback helps—but only if asked for by a teen.
- Praise privately—kids, especially teens, are hypersensitive about standing out in front of friends.
- Encourage a passion—self-confidence generalizes.
- Manners matter—rudeness to parents lowers self-esteem in kids.
- Don't "fix"—hear out a child's self-doubts.
- Encourage good deeds—action that helps others makes kids feel good about themselves.

moved on to the next thing." They needed to build on small victo-
ries that represented notable triumphs over Nan's own temperament.

By not "punctuating" modest accomplishments, parents miss
an opportunity to forge a better relationship with their adolescents. Acknowledging effort is one of the most important messages
21st-century teens need: *Try what is difficult—you will get better at it
and you will eventually feel better about yourself.*

Help Parents Create Homes Teens Love

Some parents have a relatively easy time making their house a
drop-in center for the second family. Others have to work at it. But
the end result is almost always the same: When an adolescent's
friends want to be around parents, that child becomes more recep-
tive to adult guidance. When kids hang out, they wander in and
talk to parents; parents hear bits and pieces of what is going on;
kids are relaxed and reveal more; they will ask for advice—other
people's mothers and fathers always seem "smarter" than one's
own; parents have more concrete information to guide their kids—
after all, plans and changes to plans happen with them nearby. All
of this adds up to a major shift: the wall of silence feels less formi-
dable.

The Youngs, a family I knew, seemed to handle this effort-
lessly. Starting in junior high, their house became a hotel for six to
eight kids at a time. Dora and Tom weren't the richest people, did-
n't have the nicest house, didn't even own a big entertainment center. So, what was their secret?

Their campaign began the summer before Kirk entered seventh grade. "Now that you're getting ready for junior high," they
told him, "we want to make your room into a place where you and
your friends can hang out. But we need your help." Together, the
three of them went through Kirk's things and got rid of a lot of
clutter. They built shelves and bunk beds to maximize the space,
and finally gave the room a new paint job—deep purple, a color
neither of the parents would have chosen!

The new arrangement created space for comfort time, without Dora and Tom having to compromise their standards. Whenever Kirk brought his friends around, Mom and Dad wisecracked with them, but they also acted like parents, not just buddies. As a result, everyone loved to meet and sleep over at the Youngs' house. It didn't hurt that the refrigerator was well-stocked—with junk *and* healthier food.

Dora also told Kirk's friends what she expected of them: No smoking. When you take food out of the refrigerator and don't finish it, rewrap what's left and put it back. Clean the counter after eating. If it's raining, remove your shoes at the door. In this way, the Youngs let the kids know that the adults were in charge but, at the same time, nurtured them. Whoever came to the house had to call his parents and let them know where he was—that was the price of admission. Dora and Tom were never in the kids' faces; they stayed in the next room but every once in a while popped in to say hello. While a few of Kirk's friends clung to the anonymity of hanging out in his room, more often, kids would wander into the kitchen or living room and start up conversations with his mom or dad. It was all very easy and organic. Most important, the Youngs always knew where their son was and what he was up to.

The Young's secret, then, was their ability to maintain that tricky balance, setting limits yet also knowing when to hold back. They had clear expectations of their son and his friends, but also a genuine interest in what these youngsters did and thought. I'm not surprised that even now, some 10 years later, their son Kirk, a college graduate, *still* brings other kids over during the holidays.

I learned from watching Dora and Tom that to make your house into a place kids flock to, one must be a parental presence, communicating directly with your child's friends. By telling the other boys what she expected, Dora made sure everyone knew the score, which kept her son from feeling as if he was in the middle. Imagine what a burden it is on a teen to be responsible for making friends conform to his parents' rules. It's like a child of divorce caught between warring parties, but here a child would feel torn between his two "families," the one at home and the one out there.

Comfort Time with Teens Equals Quality Time

Contrary to stereotype, teens appreciate downtime with parents. Despite their initial objections, nondemanding rituals serve as anchors in the swirl of adolescent life. Follow these guidelines with parents and they will have more success creating comfortable connections with teens.

♦ Choose an activity kids love—and parents don't hate.

♦ Make it regular, brief, and easygoing.

♦ Don't use the activity as a chance to remind, nag, or bring in worldly worries.

♦ Adapt the activity so friends can join in.

♦ Keep it brief.

♦ Become knowledgeable about the area—natural discussions will follow.

♦ Be prepared to take kids' lead in off-the-cuff conversations that the activity may trigger.

♦ Balance between regularly scheduled events, such as a shared TV program, and spontaneous ideas like a quick drive to the mall.

♦ Parallel time counts—reading alongside each other, doing paperwork and homework nearby.

♦ Bedtime rituals are still valued—try not to let a serious diagnosis, wrangling, TV, the computer, or the late hour get in the way of a kiss goodnight, a prayer, or an "I love you."

---

*   *   *

Don't let parents down—you have a lot to offer. These strategies comprise a significant body of expertise for mothers and fathers, proven by decades of clinical and longitudinal research, as well as by child and adult surveys. If parents cannot implement these approaches, it is almost always a sign of more serious pathology, a family secret, or unaddressed dynamics.

To move the process along, to change the dance, you now have to challenge yourself in a way that paralyzes so many child professionals: You may need to call for a family session. Try not to be overly worried about this. The "focused family sessions" I describe in the next chapter are manageable.

They can help you create the kind of relational–behavioral shifts that transform stalled treatment into dramatic change.

STUCK

> Ron, I don't understand it. I'm trying to find a referral for a
> friend's teenage daughter. Either they only see kids and won't
> involve the parents, or they only see families and won't see the
> kid alone. I thought we'd gotten further than this in the field.
> —*An extremely experienced professional in a major,
> urban–suburban hub*

> Slowly you turn yourself from a bridge into a well-worn path.
> Your office has become the town's center, a place where park
> benches still exist.

During the course of work with adolescents, there are times
when it is absolutely essential to meet with the family, instead
of with the child or parents alone. This is troublesome for many
therapists. For the most part, we are trained to work individually
with children or do guidance with parents or see families as a
whole. Our narrow specialization drives families crazy. Having personally done and supervised thousands of initial interviews, I've
learned that one of the biggest complaints patients have is a sense
they are being forced into the teaching model of a training facility
or the orientation of a private practitioner. This is maddening to
prospective clients—approximately half terminate prematurely and
find what they want elsewhere. Within many agencies, the family

is divided according to modality. When assigned as a "family" case, few of the treating therapists are equipped to see kids alone; if it is considered a "child" case, few of these therapists can handle the family in a room together. *Almost none can move between modalities, keeping all relationships intact.*

What a perfect metaphor: Fragmented homes, already pulled between first and second families, now find themselves in a field that replicates the disconnection that got kids into trouble in the first place. The relational–behavioral approach is a way to address this fragmentation, challenging the distance between parents and kids while strengthening both kids' and parents' competence. Paraphrasing Winnicott, the 21st-century helping professional must create a flexible container: see kids alone, see parents alone, and feel competent to conduct what I call *"focused family sessions"* when needed.

This is a difficult balancing act. In a disconnected world, however, it is necessary to integrate modalities. The information you receive from parents and kids and the way you use this information in conjoint meetings challenges family members to make significant changes in their behavior. This creates connections and family relationships previously considered impossible.

Why a Focused Family Session?

Talking in individual meetings is not enough. Dylan complains about his "crazy" mother. He describes to me how they get into fights over his grades and increasingly strident demands to go out with friends during the week. Interactions at home escalate, sometimes into physical standoffs. Recently, Dylan loomed over his mother with a baseball bat in hand, screaming he'd use it (not a real threat) if she pressed on. They are obviously stuck. When I work with Dylan alone I challenge him to make concrete changes around the house. His mother might not be so hysterical if he approached her less provocatively, or in a respectful way that eased her mind, at least slightly, about the kind of privileges he was demanding. At the same time, parent sessions did not lead to changes either. Dylan's mother, Yvette, still pounced like a tigress when he was slow to co-operate. She couldn't stop focusing on his disorganized room. Yvette exploded almost every time he pushed for a later curfew, once rushing from the bathtub naked to block him at the front door. Often, child and parent are like a dysfunctional couple who can't transfer what is discussed in the room to acting differently at home.

The inability to create individual or systemic change leads kids down a dangerous path. For example, Frederick, 14, talked at length in our sessions about his father's ferocious temper, his mother's attempts to play peacemaker, and his own efforts to stand up for himself. Frederick and I tried to figure out how he might handle these scenes in a better way. I also met with Mom and Dad, as I regularly do, to try to get them to manage anger differently. Very little shifted—family life was temporarily quiet, then new explosions always flared up.

Meanwhile, outside the house, Frederick spent more time playing at the edge of danger. Pushing the envelope, he slept around, stayed out later, drank more, and went to after-hour clubs and extremely sketchy areas of town. Frederick became unmotivated in school, which had always been a sustaining involvement. The situation was stuck. The cycle of explosion, peacemaking, remorse, truce and explosion kept recurring.

In such mired-down cases—after I have met with an adolescent for some time alone and with parent(s), separately—it is necessary to have a "focused family session" *before* a major crisis occurs.

What Are Focused Family Sessions?

Focused family sessions, as I have developed them, synthesize family systems theory, even as most sessions are individual ones with the adolescent or parents. The "focus" in focused family sessions is essential, so that the therapist can maintain control of family meetings *and* protect empathic connections with both teen and parent. Fears of unmanageable eruptions during conjoint sessions, stony silence on a teen's part, and vicious scapegoating in all directions discourage therapists from entering into this territory. In hundreds of consultations with families of adolescents, I have heard complaints by both parents and teens who say past family sessions were episodes of unprocessed venting, huge disappointments or events that shook their faith in the entire change process.

It is such a difficult balancing act to manage individual as well as family sessions, it's no wonder few training facilities offer this approach (check the brochures or websites of programs around the country).

To begin, use the following guidelines for focused family sessions:

+ The frame of the session is extremely specific—to shift a single stuck interaction or issue. Success is more attainable when the frame is limited.

+ Goals are defined ahead of time, thereby lessening surprises for kids and parents.

+ The fact that you will temporarily ally with the other "side" is predicted. This is done in order to protect empathic connections for future individual meetings.

The overarching purpose of a focused family session is to help parent(s) and teen shift one troublesome, repetitive interaction between them. That's it! The goal is not to figure out how the entire family dynamic needs to change or how each member might improve communication or how to resolve transgenerational issues, and so on.

The Choreography of Change

My narrow definition of a family session evolved from work I originally did over 20 years ago at the Philadelphia Child Guidance Clinic. I was then trained in structural family therapy with Salvador Minuchin and Virginia Goldner, and later in family systems therapy with Betty Carter. Structural family therapy teaches us that changing the interaction in one area of family life allows individuals to move beyond symptomatic behaviors; they begin to differentiate in healthier ways. Structural family therapy had its most profound impact in the '70s and '80s. It produced dramatic videotapes of sessions so charged that reestablishing empathetic connections in subsequent individual meetings would be quite a challenge.

For example, in one famous videotaped session, Mother and Father became sufficiently frustrated with their anorexic teen that they literally shoved a frankfurter down her throat—at the therapist's urgings that Mom and Dad take charge. This shocking intervention, a kind of therapeutic performance art, restructured the entire hierarchy: The sick child was no longer in charge of her parents. This girl could now begin to eat for herself, according to what these family therapists believed.

Another dramatic videotape involved a family in which the two adolescent boys were out of control—defying their parents and in trouble with police. In the taped session (considered then to be a breakthrough), Dad physically wrestled one of his teenage sons to the floor. From that session, as was the case with the anorexic girl, the family pattern significantly shifted. Kids reconstituted because parents were now in charge and the children were not.

Even then I never believed that most of the time one session had the stand-alone power to entirely rearrange the course of family life or of child development (see my article "Revolution/Evolution: Feminism Forces Us to Reconsider Our Expectations about Dramatic Cures," *The Family Therapy Networker*, 1986). Actually, I learned during my externship at Philadelphia Child Guidance how much behind-the-scenes help was offered to kids and families—individual sessions, parenting, and psychoeducational input. These important change agents were left on the cutting room floor. Not dramatic enough for audiences, but a critical part of the paradigm that I valued even more as I learned about all the quiet attention families received.

So, despite dramatic videos, one family session doesn't usually do the trick. It is truly powerful, however, if *after* a dysfunctional dance is challenged during family meetings, the therapist continues to see family members to strengthen different ways of dealing with each other. The power of structured interventions is exponentially increased when transgenerational issues can be dealt with before or after focused family sessions. Even if a specific interaction cannot be dislodged in a focused family meeting, it almost always has a transgenerational etiology that may be addressed later on. Interestingly, my training in systemic family therapy (à la Betty Carter) emphasized how work could be done in sessions in which family members talk just to the therapist in the room. These two vastly different perspectives are wonderful complements to each other—if you are able to conceive of your role as a bridge between the teen and adult worlds.

Preparing for Focused Family Sessions

In order to protect existing empathic connections, it is necessary to prepare both adolescent and parent for a focused family session. Once a family interaction gets underway, each "side" can feel totally abandoned by you. The family format seems strange to clients used to seeing you alone. The empathic connection of the private session is now fraught with potential for you to be experienced as favoring the other. In addition, clients often land in your office because of out-of-control dynamics. Naturally, both parent and teen are afraid (or secretly hope) that similar escalations will take place in the family meeting: "Now, you'll really see how crazy my mother is; now you'll finally understand how impossible my kid is." They're often right; family sessions can get wildly out of control, so I prepare in the following ways:

♦ *First, define ahead of time exactly what the topic will be.* To one boy and his parents I said: "We're going to talk about curfews— nothing more." To a girl and her mother I said, "The topic is going to be the fights in the morning about what clothes you're wearing. That's it." At the beginning of the family session, I remind both what we'll be talking about. It's important to limit the scope in this way. John Gottman, noted researcher on the "science of communication," (*Observing Interaction*, 1997) is right. Relationship fights are so volatile, they instantaneously move into a physiologically inflamed laundry list of hot-button issues.

♦ *At the start of the session, remind both parents and kids that they will probably feel unhappy about your role.* I say to my teen client, "Listen, at some point during this meeting you're going to feel I'm taking your parent's side. Don't worry. It's just temporary, to find what works better for you and them." To parent(s): "At some point, you're going to feel like I'm taking your child's side against you. It's for the purpose of moving the session ahead. Try to remember that I'm not abandoning your perspective."

♦ *Remind everyone that whatever happens during the session, you will have a chance to talk in private meetings.* This "to-be-continued" approach takes the heat off everyone, including professionals, and it is the truth. No one should enter a focused family session worrying that it will make or break the relationship. This is the therapeutic equivalent of that mythical "birds and bees" discussion about sex. In real 21st-century life such sex-talks rarely happen just once; rather, minidiscussions on the topic occur many times over. In the same way, real change usually occurs over time. For focused family sessions to work, the hope for instant transformation needs to be lessened, or disappointment is sure to follow.

Enactments and Focused Family Sessions

The specific structural technique to use in focused family sessions is "the enactment." Family members, if prodded to discuss a conflictual issue, invariably act out their most important dynamics. While we all may not have been formally taught this principle, we are certainly familiar with it. Enactments happen in our lives all the time. Borrowed originally from interpersonal psychoanalytic theory, "enactment" is another way to say that family communicational patterns are so ingrained they spontaneously appear no matter how determined we are to avoid them.

♦ *Foster an interaction between parents and child over a stuck issue, previously identified in individual sessions.* The topic must be one that is currently "alive" to all parties. It may be curfew, friends, verbal abuse, drugs, alcohol, back talk, homework, keeping the room clean, how parents and kids listen to each other, and so on. Your goal is to start parent and child talking to each other (not to you) about one concrete issue. For example, you might say, "Discuss with your son the chores you'd like done. This is an area you've all described as a problem." The authority with which you can lead is the relational traction you've gained from previous sessions with parent and teen alone.

♦ *Prepare family members for a moment or two of self-consciousness.* Even if they have known you for years, most people are self-conscious when asked to discuss personal matters in front of a non-family member. Awkwardness needs to be addressed. Say, "This will seem strange at first. But I guarantee in a few minutes, it will feel much more natural." Normalize by referring to the many other experiences you've had with enactments (remember, in your personal as well as professional life these interactions go on all the time). Or, if you can't think of specific examples, be honest and say, "I'd like to try a technique I've just learned."

♦ *To start the interaction, make yourself as invisible as possible.* There are several ways to do this. Don't make eye contact with family members, since this leads to greater self-consciousness. How? Lean back, literally face another direction, or look down at your notes. The boundary expressed through your body language communicates that whatever goes on is the *family's* doing, not an artificial exchange created by being in your presence.

After it gets going, artificial as it may feel or as much as a parent or child initially objects—the strength of the "dance" is so powerful you're quickly into the thick of it. Whenever one has a strong relationship—and what is more intense than a parent–teen showdown—the interaction gets going almost exactly the way it happens around the house. *As you listen, your role changes.*

A Quick Enactment Guide

Observe the most concrete behaviors, the basic steps in the family's dance. Don't look for hidden motivation. Ask yourself questions that begin with words such as "what," "who," and "where." Do not get yourself stuck on asking "why" or "when." The following are some examples of what to look for.

♦ *Tone of voice*—respectful, contemptuous, and so forth. A nice-guy dad complains that his boy, James, is an inexplicable wise guy in school. Mom is also concerned about her son's negative attitude with other adults, with whom he constantly finds fault. During the enactment, this very nice man surprisingly speaks to his son in a derisive tone, especially when the boy disagrees with him. "I've never heard anything so ridiculous," he says. Dad's attitude infuriates his son and, in turn, the boy shouts, "Yeah? . . . You don't know anything either!" further aggravating the father.

♦ *Loudness*—Who drowns out whom? In the Marion family, everyone had to yell to be heard. Katie, a fifth grader who had trouble standing up for herself in school, was unable to speak during the enactment. As everyone screamed at each other over every possible issue, Katie could not get a word in edgewise. In just a few minutes, it was clear where she had learned to be so reserved.

♦ *Reactivity*—the quickness and intensity of family members' responses to each other. Parents had complained about disagreements over the kids. They then demonstrated their endless fighting when the counselor got them to discuss a time for the next appointment. They were so inflamed that the counselor told me, "It was as if I didn't exist in the room."

♦ *Listening*—Who listens? Who does not? Dad was a wonderful listener while the family discussed differences of opinion. Mom, on the other hand, lectured to their oppositional and sullen daughter. The more Dad listened, the more Mom said he was being too soft-hearted and launched into another lecture. During this interaction, Mom, who was just as concerned about her daughter's welfare, became "the bad guy" compared to ever-patient dad.

♦ *Relatedness*—Who's talking to whom? Who's left out? A tough-guy father interrupted loudly and repeatedly barged into the conversation I got going about curfew for his adolescent son. Despite his ineffectiveness, Dad prided himself on being the family's teacher of life lessons. As the enactment went on, this tough guy was slowly pushed to the periphery. No one talked about anything without going through Mom; certainly no one listened to Dad as he barked and sputtered from the sidelines.

♦ *Leadership*—Who speaks first? In some families, the person who speaks first during the enactment is a paper tiger. In others, this person sets the tone of the entire discussion. The latter was the case in the Johnson family. Whatever mood Dad was in seemed to set the stage for any discussion that followed. Enactments were merely a reflection of dad's predominant mood.

♦ *Closure*—Who gets in the last word? Can a conclusion be reached? With Annie, a 14-year-old who was in trouble because of acting out in school, the enactment between her and her mom was very telling: Annie always had to get the last word in. Unfortunately, so did her mother. Keeping the enactments down to several minutes was next to impossible since, just like at home, they could never end their arguments. Each just got madder at the other and more determined to have the last world.

Empathic Punctuation

♦ *Punctuation is your empathic feedback about the dance parent and child get caught up in.* While not originally presented in this way by structural family therapists, punctuation reestablishes the empathic connections you have spent individual sessions creating, connections you may temporarily lose during the heat of the family's exchange. This eye on empathic traction, while pushing for change, is essential in a relational–behavioral approach.

Here are some illustrations:

Fifteen-year-old Amy and her mother Jolie came to a focused family session. I had been seeing both in individual sessions for several months. The troublesome issues for this mother had to do with her daughter's staying out late and being maddeningly secretive. I said, "Amy, talk to your mom about having a later curfew." Immediately, their interaction made it clear that Jolie was intensely provoked by Amy's silence or obfuscations. Mom began communicating with her daughter primarily by asking a lot of demanding questions. Of course, the more she grilled Amy, the more her daughter clammed up. Amy became deeply sullen and, if possible, even less present.

When the nature of the interaction is clear, you can punctuate—offer feedback to both sides. In this case, I said, "Amy, you have a lot more power over your mother than *you or I* may have realized. Your clamming up is driving Mom crazy and getting her to ask one question after another." To Mom: *"Now I understand even better* how your frustration makes you want to pull your hair out— but endless questions don't seem to be getting you anywhere."

Another example: In our private meetings, Dylan complained that his mother, Yvette, "got hysterical" when things weren't done her way. Mom repeatedly complained how stubborn her adolescent son was: "It's like talking to a brick wall." So, when individual sessions didn't change the dance, I called for a focused family session. I asked Dylan and Yvette to talk about keeping his room neater, a conflict both had separately mentioned. As they started interacting, it became immediately clear that Mom jumped into sweeping generalizations, "If you can't keep your room clean, if you don't have that kind of basic sense of responsibility, what does that say about your whole character? As you get older, how are you going to maintain a job? Any boss you have isn't going to stand for this." Dylan, in turn, was no slouch. He became sharply belligerent, calling her almost every name he could think of—"You're a lunatic. You're crazy. You're worse than any parent I've ever met. You get absolutely insane over these stupid little things." In the way he talked to her, he *became* exactly what she had accused him of being—thoughtless and irresponsible.

Empathic punctuation: Mother and son needed to see what they were doing in this exchange. I said, "Mom, you're letting Dylan get you so upset, *I can really see how* his whole future is flashing before your eyes. Dylan, the more you keep calling your mother names about how "off the wall" she gets, the angrier she becomes. *Soon, she'll be grounding you for life.*"

The point about punctuation is that you must *empathically* address each participant. In the dance that is taking place, point out both parent's and teen's behavior. This is a departure from traditional structural family therapy. We were trained to *unbalance* stuck dances, the idea being that with enough pressure—repetition, directives, urging, even shaming—some family member would change a step in the dance. In focused family sessions, however, you are a bridge, and maintaining empathic balance is incredibly important. You need to hold the connection with family members who have come to trust you in individual sessions. You need to think about future sessions, protecting what you've already built.

♦ *Address different family members with respect.* Try not to sound authoritarian or, especially, act the part of the self-important professional. This is easier said than done. After all, a lot of family therapy arose from an era informed by Harry Stack Sullivan and the supervisees of Eric Fromm, the interpersonal psychoanalyst. Therapists were expected to decisively "nail" people with precise interpretations. (Actually, Salvador Minuchin himself was quite a contradiction. I've met several of his ex-patients, who uniformly commented on his brilliance *and* empathic kindness toward them—"What a nice guy," each fondly remembered.)

Many professionals, however, still don't realize their legacy and have a hard time keeping away from flashy but subtly disrespectful communication. This is especially important if you are going to resume individual sessions after a focused family meeting. Provocative pronouncements such as "Your child has you wrapped around her finger" may be true, but the humiliation and shame such statements create can rupture a parent's relationship with you.

I learned this lesson years ago. Once, sitting with a family, I

was struck that during the enactment each person seemed to protect the feelings of another family member. Instead of commenting
on how sensitive they were toward each other, I came up with
the pithy observation that their exchange reminded me of the
way communication might sound in a well-mannered "protection
racket." This was right on the money, but it was delivered in a curt,
sarcastic tone that severed my connection with the family.

Such statements make for dramatic showmanship and temporary satisfaction about being tough, but they often mark the last
time we will see a family. Compare the statement "Your child has
you wrapped around her finger" with "Your child is incredibly tenacious. It's no wonder that she has you wrapped around her finger." Direct but balanced feedback is exactly what helps family
members continue to feel understood. It prepares them for the
idea that change is about *everyone working on something*. In this
case, after commenting on the child's tenacity, it's easier to move
toward directives that will be experienced empathically: "Since
your daughter is so tenacious, we need to figure out ways that can
help you to be more in charge. Because of her strong will, you
might have to work harder than other parents." I will never just say
to Mother, "You're acting in a way that's ineffective," or to a teen,
"You're being absolutely dismissive of your parent"—without tying
each remark, in some way, to the other's place in the interaction.

Keep in mind the following rules about feedback:

♦ The problem is almost never one person's fault.

♦ You are not blaming anyone as being single-handedly responsible for difficult interactions.

♦ You do your best to see the situation from everyone's point
of view.

♦ Each person is part of a system that is interdependent—
therefore everyone has to change a little.

The better the balance, the more both parent and child can
stay connected to you and move on to the next step in the ses-

Empathic Feedback That Gets Through

Unbalanced	Balanced
"You don't understand your child."	"Your child is challenging and complicated. It's not surprising how difficult she is to understand."
"You're yelling at your parents too much."	"Your mom's stubborn, but yelling doesn't seem to be getting through, either."
"You criticize your child a lot of the time."	"I know you're frustrated and that easily turns into criticism; it's difficult to know what to do with him in the moment."
"You need to listen better to your parents."	"It's always hard when there are two tough parents like these. You'll have to learn to listen to one at a time."
"As his parents, you've got to be more of a united team."	"Your family's so busy, it's just about impossible for the two of you to discuss and think through decisions. . . . "
"Your father's not crazy, you just have him wrapped around your finger."	"Your father does get a little crazy; in part it's because you know exactly which buttons to push."

sion—figuring out how to do something, just one thing, a little differently.

Moving Toward Change

Create small change. Focused family sessions are not about change on a grand scale. Rather, I push both adolescent and parent to alter a very specific aspect of the dance. I want to challenge each in the session. And, à la Salvador Minuchin (also, let's not forget our strategic family therapy heritage—Haley, Madanes, Hoffman, and others), change in the moment can sometimes be the beginning of change in the entire family system.

Most child professionals I have supervised ask people to take steps that are simply too big. We push them to be different from who they are; we forget belief systems that predate us and extend way into the past. Sadly, we do all this primarily because many of us suffer from a kind of "clinical narcissism." Too many of us have the view that clients exist only in the moments we see them. I experienced this painful phenomenon first-hand when one of our children needed to be evaluated. He endured, as did we, an "arena evaluation." After an hour observing him, the team was ready to make their final, life-altering suggestions about our son. It was a traumatizing and enlightening experience, one which I described in an article in *The Psychotherapy Networker* ("Honoring the Everyday," 1995).

Supervisors of family therapy would watch 30 seconds of a session and draw sweeping conclusions about parents' entire character structure. Because of this tradition, it may be hard to imagine what people are like when we're not around. Especially with difficult parents, the complexity of everyday family life often eludes us: The family has more loving aspects than we can possibly imagine, or deals with more extraordinary adversity than we can immediately understand.

To create change means that we see mothers and fathers accurately enough so that we do not ask too much (or too little) of them. This relational-attunement is necessary to transform a difficult parent into one whose mind is open enough that new behavior is possible. Here are a number of examples taken from focused family sessions in which I pushed for small changes from both teen and parent, while trying to maintain connections throughout. My comments are always informed by what I have learned during private sessions before, and the awareness of needing to reestablish meetings afterwards.

Challenging Kids

Dylan talked to his mother in starkly disrespectful ways—making her even "crazier." I said: "Dylan, I know how important it is to you to sound older—*the kids in your grade are merciless toward anyone who sounds reasonable*—but, I don't think you're getting through to your mother. In fact, it makes her so upset she treats you more like a child. If you want to get what you want, and I think you do, you need to talk without calling her names."

In this way, I respected Dylan's context, but asked him to experiment with different way of speaking, not because it was morally right (though I believe it was), but because his behavior ensured not getting what he wanted.

Frederick, the adolescent who was inching ever closer toward dangerous behavior, taunted his father, Jack, when he reacted contemptuously about Frederick's choice of friends. In a family session, Frederick responded to his father's objections with comments like "You've got a problem," "You're old," "You can't understand anything I say about my friends anyway," "I wish I had another father," "You don't belong in this family." It was no surprise that Jack could not help but react aggressively. Veins in his neck and his forehead bulged. Deeply hurt, Dad's reaction was to become even more aggressive. Then Frederick paid even less attention to what he was saying.

I gave Frederick this challenge: "It's hard for me to ask you to forgive your dad's temper, *but remember I'm on your side here*. Even so, I want you to talk to him in such a way that you sound *like the good friend you can be to others*, and not like a child who's having a tantrum"

Reminding Frederick what a truly good person he could be to his friends assured Frederick that I was not abandoning him. This allowed me to bluntly challenge him to change his steps in the dance.

* * *

Rice, the girl who refused to take a shower and was increasingly belligerent in school, came to a family session with her mother. At home, battles erupted nightly. Rice adamantly defended why she shouldn't have to bathe—the teacher said they didn't have to shower that much, few of her friends took many showers, and so forth. Her mother's response to these excuses was something like "You get dirty and smelly. I don't want to live in a house with somebody who takes a shower only once a week," and so on. The arguments always escalated, sometimes accompanied by near-physical confrontations.

Talking about showers in a focused family session might sound like a silly issue for treatment, but the violent interaction these two got into was no small matter. It was important to challenge each to approach this "dance of anger" (Harriet Lerner, 1985) differently.

I said to Rice: "I know you don't want to take a shower every night. *I know how much you can't stand getting your skin wet, how sensitive it is.* But, it seems like the more excuses you make, the more insistent your mom gets about the whole thing, *and you know how stubborn your mother can be.* You need to listen to her for a minute, without coming up with an excuse." This was my challenge to Rice—to be quiet, if just for a few seconds. I protected our empathic connection by validating her experience of Mom being an incredibly strong-willed, rigid person. I used the information from private sessions to stay connected with Rice, even as I pushed her to change.

Alvin wanted to drive the family car. His father, Arnold, believed Alvin wouldn't be entirely truthful about very serious issues: whether he would drive while drinking; whether he would chauffeur other kids around, even if he was too tired or drunk; and how fast would he drive. His fear was understandable, inflamed by the recent deaths of four neighborhood kids when, after a keg party, one of the boys wrapped the car around a tree. In talking about all this, Alvin attempted to be Mr. Smooth, coming up with superficially clever, made-for-TV arguments: "Well, you know I never touch a drink during the week, so I don't know why you'd worry about me driving. I can give you my full-faith, absolute, sacred guarantee: There's no way I'd touch an ounce of liquor if I'm out with the car."

To this, Arnold would reply: "How can you say that? What difference do the weekdays make? You're going to parties on the weekends all the time; I know you go to bars with other kids. How can you promise you'll never touch anything?" Alvin responded with 10 reasons why such a situation was completely ludicrous. Drinking during the week showed real alcohol dependence, so obviously, he didn't have a problem; his friends looked out for each other—they didn't want him to get busted, and on and on. The more he tried to "sell" these ideas, the more nervous dad got.

In trying to change Alvin's part of the interaction, I presented this challenge: "Alvin, you're sounding like a potentially successful lawyer. *I have faith that one day you're going to make tons of money.* But can you see that the more you try to *impress* your father with these arguments, the less he seems to trust you? So, what I'd like you to do is talk more slowly. Give yourself and him time to think." Previous sessions with Alvin helped me understand his deep desire to succeed, to make big bucks, and to impress. Clearly, I used this empathic grasp, even as I pushed him to drop the "con artist" façade.

* * *

Ruth, 13½, wanted to go to a loft party. The precursors to "raves," loft parties typically involve several hundred teens with absolutely no adult supervision. Kids arrive from all parts of town and pay a cover charge to have unfettered access to each other and free-flowing substances. The more Ruth's parents asked her about the party, the more vague she became. Ruth would not say where it was, who was going, when it would end, and so on. I said: "Ruth, the vaguer you are, *the less chance you'll get to go to this party or others that I know are coming up.* Even though I like you so much, I'm not sure I'd even let you go, and it's clear that your parents are getting more and more upset. *You want them to trust you about a lot of things,* so you're going to have to be more specific about the details of what's involved." My appeal to Ruth was to understand her desire for greater privileges, which she'd expressed many times in our sessions. I could completely side with her parents about this party, as long as I recognized her need to be treated in a more mature, trusting way.

Challenging Parents

In troubled families, the dance is dysfunctional from both sides of the generational divide. Obviously, parents need to be pushed. Here are ways I challenged parents in three of the enactments described earlier. Again, keep in mind the importance of maintaining an empathic connection, so individual meetings in the future will still be possible.

To Dylan's "insane, hysterical" mother, I said: *"As a parent, I totally understand your frustration.* But you do sound hysterical, *like we get at home with our kids. I know it's hard, because you'd like the automatic respect your own parents got.* I'm asking you to lower your voice, though. Speak softer and a little lower—let's see what happens." My identification as a "fellow traveler," another harried parent of a 21st-century teen, was not lost on Dylan's mother who secretly believed she was an ineffective mess, totally to blame for her son's difficulties.

*   *   *

Frederick's father, Jack, became so agitated while talking to his son, he visibly stiffened in his seat. He got up, and began looming over Frederick in a physically intimidating way. At that point I said: *"We know each other so well by now. When Frederick talks to you, I can almost feel your reactions.* Pay attention to how much your whole body is starting to tense up. As Frederick talks, try to be aware of your body. *It's a simple exercise many parents of teenagers need to learn.* The more aggressive you get, the more disrespectful and babyish he's going to behave. And, *I know from your history that's not what you want for Frederick."* Again, meeting with Jack several times before this session gave legitimacy to my empathic remarks. I did know him well. I knew how hurt he was beneath that aggressive stance and how much he wanted to avoid the decades-long estrangement he had endured with his own father.

*   *   *

To Rice's mother, I said: "Arlene, *everyone, including me, admires how quick your mind is and how logical you are.* But rational arguments aren't working. I want you to try to talk to Rice without using logic to convince her. Use your imagination. Cut a deal if you have to. *I know how creative you can be in your work negotiations."* In sessions before this enactment, I had many times commented on Arlene's intellectual acuity. Arlene didn't let my challenge upset here because she truly believed I admired her tenacity. This empathic recognition enabled her to take my suggestion seriously, without rupturing our connection.

Putting It Together

Following are summaries of extended dialogues from two of the families described earlier. In them you will recognize the basic principles of a focused family session: protecting and referring back to already established relationships, pushing for very specific change, aiming for greater effectiveness in family members—all the while nurturing your connection for subsequent private sessions.

*   *   *

FREDERICK: (*to Jack, his father*) You're a real bully! Why are you always pushing Mom around like that? You're always bossing her.

DAD: Well, it's my right. You're not married to her, I am. When you get married, then you can treat your wife the way you want to. Anyway, *she's* not complaining.

FREDERICK: I'll never be like you. I can't stand the way you act. I hate the way you are around the house.

Jack, upset and angry, starts to get out of his chair and walk over to where Frederick is sitting. The scene looks threatening. Mom starts to rise at the same time, moving to block her husband from going over to Frederick.

THERAPIST: (*to Mom*) I know how you worry, but please, Sherry, let them handle this. "Frederick, you can say whatever you want outside this room. But I want you to try to talk to your father another way here. *I know the many ways you talk so well in other situations.* I want you to try to speak toward him in a way that doesn't sound like a *disrespectful* kid who's just trying to get his goat. And Jack, I'd like you to move back. *Frederick isn't a little boy anymore, the one you miss so much, even though he sounds like one right now.* Standing over him, it seems as if you're trying to remind him that you're still Big Daddy. I'd like you to talk to Frederick in a way where you don't have to stand up over him.

A long pause follows. Not a word is said. Jack is back in his seat; Frederick sits glowering. Eventually they speak again:

FREDERICK: When you stand over me like that, I forget everything good you ever did for me. All I do is hate you.

DAD: Yeah, like you ever remember anything I do for you in the first place!

THERAPIST: Frederick, what you just said now sounded different from the way you were talking before, *more like the way you've described other relationships to me.* Jack, I see you're getting upset again. I want you to try to calm yourself down. You don't have to be so big. *Talk to Frederick from the quieter side you've shared with me privately.*

DAD: All right . . . all right . . . all right. (*With each "all right," Jack seems to be calming himself down. Then, in a lower voice:*) Frederick, what do you mean when you say that? [This is the first time Jack has ever asked his son to clarify what he's talking about.]

FREDERICK: Well, I hate you so much that I forget you do a lot of things for me. (*At this point, Frederick's eyes fill up.*)

DAD: Like what?

FREDERICK: Like, you're the only father who drives me and my friends around all the time, and brings us places. Mostly mothers do it, but you bring me to my friend's houses.

DAD: You always treated me like the chauffeur. I never knew it mattered to you or that you even noticed.

THERAPIST: Frederick, it's true, you can manipulate your father and make him feel useless. *Even though I know what he does secretly matters to you.*

FREDERICK: (*smiling wearily*) Well, I know how I can get to him.

THERAPIST: Jack, you stand up and try to display your raw power. It's almost like you're challenging Frederick to fight you. Please talk to him about your anger, *like you've talked to me about it before.*

DAD: (*thinking for a long while*) I want you to be tougher. I don't want you to get scared. I want you to stand up to people. I almost wish you'd stand up and just, you know, clock me one. So, I could feel like I did my job, that I made you tough enough for the world out there. (*long pause; again in a lower voice*) Frederick, I love you. I just wish you didn't make me so mad.

Frederick is annoyed by this last comment from Jack (because Dad's blaming *him* for Dad's own anger). He starts to get provocative again. They're suddenly at the edge of another physical fight; Dad moves forward in his seat, Mom moves forward in hers.

THERAPIST: Jack, just keep talking. Don't move forward. You caught it and controlled it just in time. You were about to get up. *I know how well you can work with people.* You don't have to use raw muscle power to make Frederick tougher. And, Frederick, *with the way friends respect you,* you don't have to keep provoking your dad just to prove that you can push him around.

FREDERICK: Dad, I don't want to push my girlfriend around the way you do us. And you know what? I don't want to work all the time, like you do. I wish that you would just listen to things I say to you, instead of worrying about making me tougher. I wish you would take just a couple of minutes to listen, without feeling you have to teach me to become like you.

JACK: You think I work too much? . . . I never said a word to my own father. He never said much to me. I barely saw him around the house, and, when he did talk to me, he was always teaching me, too. Trying to toughen me up, I guess.

FREDERICK: (*in response to his father's frankness about his own youth*) I know I make you feel like you're a servant. I take Mom's side on purpose just to get you crazy. I can't say I'm never going to do all that again. Maybe if you just stop trying to teach me all the time to be the way you think I should be, maybe I could feel a little different about you.

It's quiet in the room now. Keep in mind how many times I've referred back to our private meetings, how much I've pushed, while protecting empathic connections. Frederick and his father are looking down. Nothing dramatic happens. Jack doesn't get upset; he's just nodding. Mom looks almost relaxed, for the first time. We can all feel the change from the beginning of this interaction. Father and son are talking to each other and listening in a slightly different way.

This was a focused challenge for each to change a step of a destructive dance; and, their connection to me has survived the meeting.

*   *   *

Jolie, a single mother, is raising her youngest child alone. Amy is a junior in high school and is supposed to be thinking about college. The family has very little money and careful planning will be necessary. But, meanwhile, Amy's close to failing in school. She's dyed her hair jet black, gotten her tongue pierced, adopted a new Goth look, and become part of a wild crowd. In addition, she's coming home later and later, some nights not at all. The live issue around which I focus the enactment is curfew.

JOLIE: No matter what, I still love you. But why do you get into so much trouble all the time? I don't understand you. You promise me you'll be home by 2:00, and then there's this big excuse when you show up hours later.

AMY: Yeah, well, if you paid more attention to me you would understand what's going on.

JOLIE: What are you talking about? I do everything for you. I always ask you questions about your friends and what goes on in school and about your work. But you don't answer me.

THERAPIST: You're not getting through to each other. Amy, *I know you're great at having your own mind and doing things your own way.* Jolie, *you've always been terrific at plugging ahead in life, despite the obstacles.* But you're clearly not getting through. Try again.

JOLIE: You're always so busy. You never have time to talk, anyway.

AMY: Well, I *am* busy, because I don't want to turn into a slug like you.

JOLIE: (*very defensive*) What are you talking about, a slug! I do plenty! (*She reels off a long list of things she does for the house, for Amy, for herself.*)

THERAPIST: Jolie, you defend yourself so quickly. *It's not necessary after what you've accomplished with your life.* I don't think you deserve going on the defensive like this. And Amy, you've developed that glare into an art form! It's so perfect, you could be on MTV with it. (*Amy smirks at this.*) Go back to talking about your curfew. Jolie, try not to be so defensive. Amy, see if you can cut out the glare for a minute, no 10 seconds.

AMY: Well, look, Mom, you're so dull, nothing ever goes on around the house. So sure, I want to be with my friends. (*Jolie says nothing.*) If I go away to college, what are you going to do? You don't have a life, what are *you* going to do? (*another long pause*)

JOLIE: Well, it will be hard. It's been just the two of us for a long time. I try to show an interest and ask her questions, but she doesn't answer and she flares up at me.

THERAPIST: Jolie, you're sounding the same as before. Try to talk in a way that doesn't sound so defensive. And Amy, you've got that glare on your face again—and I know your mother secretly matters to you.

AMY: I think you want me home early because you're so bored, because you don't have your own life. It's not for any other reasons, it's not for all those things you say, like my safety. You know the group I'm in. They're not as wild as they seem. Nobody's ever gotten into bad trouble. Nobody's been arrested. Nobody's even been hurt. You just want me around the house for you.

THERAPIST: OK, Jolie, I understand this is hard. *But I've heard a lot about your life in our meetings, a lot more than you're saying to your daughter here.*

JOLIE: (*with a burst of feeling*) OK. You know what? I like it when you're here. But to be honest—and I don't want to hurt your feelings—here's the truth: I also like it when you're gone. It's *me* time. I can focus on *me*. It's quiet, I play the music *I* like, I watch *my* shows. I don't just think about you. So, if I'm going to be honest, sometimes it's OK when you're not home. . . . *In fact, I actually look forward to it.*

AMY: (*The glare on her face suddenly disappears. She gets tears in her eyes.*) But you always act like you don't have a life at all.

JOLIE: You're right, I don't have as much of a life as I'd like. But I'm not shriveling up either. And I feel like I'm actually starting to get one, a life, I mean.

THERAPIST: Can you tell Amy more about how you'll do when

she leaves, actually *if* she leaves—some of what you've shared with me. Amy, see if you can listen without interrupting or staring her down.

JOLIE: You're worried I won't make it if you go off to college.

AMY: (*after a long pause*) You're right. I think you're going to get sick. Or maybe you'll just sit around and not do anything. I bring the only life to this house. If I leave, you'll turn into a nothing.

JOLIE: (*clearly thinking hard*) Look, Amy, I can't promise you how I'm going to feel. But in my heart, I know I'm going to survive. I've been through much worse. And, I'm going to be OK. (*Amy looks skeptical.*)

THERAPIST: I'm very familiar with Amy's skepticism, I don't think she really believes you.

JOLIE: Listen, I've been through the divorce. I had no job. I got a job. I went back to school and I got a degree. The business closed down and I found another job. (*She's now crying.*) I'm going to make it, no matter what happens with you. You've got to stop worrying about me!

For the first time, Amy is listening with rapt attention. I can see she's taking it in. The "truths" that I'd learned from individual sessions were now in the space between them.

The Focused Family Session: Loose Ends

♦ *If the troublesome interaction changes within the first few minutes, the meeting can end*. Don't feel you must fill up a 45-minute or a one-hour session. Your goal is to change the choreography, to alter the interaction around one specific issue—because that one change could help parent or child relate differently to each other.

♦ *Predict "normal" setbacks after the session*. Say, "The way you were the past few minutes sounds different. But, remember, you'll probably go back to your old way of doing things. This dance has been going on for a long time. At least in the room today, you were able to do it differently for a few minutes."

♦ *Take what you saw during the enactment—what worked better and what underlying patterns emerged—and use them in private sessions afterward.* Frederick, for example, needed to work on not being provocative. (This happened not just toward his father; Frederick often antagonized friends around him.) Amy's secret caretaking of Mother was her *modus operandi* within the second family. Amy continuously fretted about whether a friend was going to stay with a boyfriend, or whether another friend was getting too deeply into drugs. Her reflexive caretaking was getting in the way of academic demands and her own needs with peers.

The experience together stays alive for future private sessions, and creates ongoing challenges for each side afterwards.

* * *

Focused family sessions close a circle. Do you remember the special sense of familiarity with old friends, whose parents you also knew as a child? That "neighborhood" feeling is exactly what happens when you bring everyone together. You've immersed yourself with teens in their world; you've immersed yourself with parents in their concerns. Now, during a focused family session, you've immersed yourself in both sides of the generational divide.

Slowly, you've turned yourself from a bridge into a well-worn path. Your office has become the town's center, a place where park benches still exist, a place where parents and children, despite all their struggles, can still come to be with each other.

10

THE VILLAGE

Bringing Friends into Treatment

The wildly successful TV show *Friends* ran for 10 years, 238 episodes, and reached million of viewers, mostly teens and preteens. It has been released on DVD and is in syndication, currently appearing several times a day nationwide, with absolutely no end in sight.

The gang from *Friends* would say "Of course!" But a controversial aspect of the model I propose is inviting the friends of your client into meetings. This is a complex issue for obvious ethical, legal, and clinical reasons. *Before using what I suggest here, be sure to speak to your supervisor or professional state agency.* Whatever you decide, I have discovered that, when appropriate, opening up the room to friends can be incredibly valuable.

It took me years before I grasped how essential it is to occasionally meet those second-family members who have just as much influence as the first family at home. My experience with Frank proved to be the tipping point. Frank was a 15-year-old boy I had been seeing for about half a year. He came to our meetings a bit early, and I noticed that his friend Dan was usually with him in the waiting room. Being a little slow on the uptake, several months passed before it dawned on me that repeatedly bringing his friend along was probably not an accident. Maybe the two planned to do something together after our session. Or, just maybe, Frank might like me to meet this friend, but, never having been trained in this matter, I didn't know what to do. One day I finally asked Frank if he'd like Dan to come in for a minute and say hello. Frank replied, "Absolutely!" Dan immediately jumped up and the three of us went into my office.

At that moment it clicked for me. Thinking about other teens I was seeing, I realized how often they, too, arrived with friends in tow. In addition, almost every therapist I knew reported the same phenomenon, specifically when working with *adolescents*—elementary school age kids rarely, if ever, bring in their friends. For a variety of reasons, we don't address the clear message: "I want you to meet the people whom I consider to be my second family." Yet for most of these teen tagalongs, that is exactly the point. During much of treatment clients are more consciously concerned about the members of their second family than the one at home. Ignoring this phenomenon represents a significant loss to the richness of treatment and our understanding of a teenager.

Some Ethical/Legal Questions to Consider

1. Must you tell the parents of your client that you have seen his friends?

2. Who pays for a meeting with a friend?

3. Are you required to tell the parent of the friend that a meeting occurred?

4. Must you inform parents immediately?

5. How long can you see a friend without changing the nature of the relationship?

6. What are your responsibilities, if you discover through a meeting, that a friend is in danger? Or is a danger to others?

Enter the Second Family

We mental health professionals have not kept pace with several decades of massive social upheaval. The world of an adolescent is now so powerfully defined by forces other than home—the peer network and pop culture—that working exclusively with your client and his or her first family is rarely powerful enough to effect change in the life of a troubled teenager.

Today's child has more than likely already been pried out of the family long before adolescence by the grasping tentacles of the pop culture. At a time when *external* forces—peer groups and mass culture—are at least as powerful in defining the adolescent's world as the *internal* family, the first family at home often exerts less pull on a teen than the second family of the peer group. For helping professionals, the consequences of this shift are enormous; we can no longer focus only on the first family in the therapy room.

Not only is the second family at least as influential as the primary family in an adolescent's life, it is likely to be just as dysfunctional. First, consider the values expressed in the role models and fads of pop culture—anorexically thin teenage fashion models; endless consumerism; hypersexualized, violence-saturated entertainment; and an ethic of sophistication that makes kids seem old before their time.

Second, since the peer group is essentially rudderless, it exemplifies Murray Bowen's undifferentiated ego mass. Once *in* the group, some individuals have trouble developing their own independent interest and values; if the old family hierarchy kept adolescents from ever leaving home, the new second family discourages them from going home. This is especially so, not in high school, as many think, but in the pressure-riddled middle school years.

Finally, like the alcoholic or abusive parent who controls a dysfunctional family, a teen leader—often one of the most disturbed kids in the group—may set the behavior patterns for the rest. This is, of course, nothing new. Young people have always admired charismatic group leaders. But today (as described in Chapter 1), the stakes are much higher. Instead of showing other kids how to inhale cigarettes, a 13-year-old might well be introducing them to smoking pot and now, increasingly, heroin; instead of making fun of an unpopular teacher, a 15-year-old will use his charm and verbal wit to get other kids to spend the night spray-painting graffiti on the sides of the school building, creating bomb scares (I've spoken to many guidance counselors on their cell phones, during school evacuations), or engaging in life-threatening sexual behavior. Many of the "shocking surprises" professionals share with me during workshops are the *modus operandi* behaviors of a second family leader.

Usually, though, we will see not this charismatic leader of the peer group, but another, less socially skilled, adolescent who plays the traditional role of the "symptom bearer" for the second family. In these cases, it may be critical that professionals not only take into account the second family, but actually bring in the leaders, if possible. The question is—how? Since I ask every child I see (first grade and up) to help me draw a "friends" sociogram, I know something about their influence and also the kinds of problems group leaders are having in their own lives.

Talking to an adolescent's friends opens up doors about how other kids see him, about the identity he has in the second family. I gain a deeper insight into who an adolescent is simply by doing what I suggest to parents all the time—make your place a home that kids feel comfortable coming to and hanging out in. In the same way, my office becomes a welcoming place for an adolescent to bring his friends. And, I can stay in closer contact with the everyday dramas of their lives.

How to Bring in Peers

Most professionals sense its importance, but have not been trained to deal with the second family and do not quite know how to approach it. Following are some ways.

FIND OUT WHO BELONGS

Therapists rarely meet the leader of the peer group: the "queen bee," the "mean girl," or the *"real-boy" bully.* Rather, it is the less socially skilled adolescent who gets "busted." In most cases, it is critical to learn about missing family members. The sociogram, then, immediately identifies second-family topography. It creates a baseline of "first names," friends whose importance and issues change almost weekly in a teen's very busy other family. It is fascinating to see how kids remind me of changes in their second family. Erin says, "You remember Xavier? The one you drew close to me? He's moving away soon, and I don't know what's going to happen to our group."

Molly says, "Let me see the map—it changed this week."

BE DIRECT: ASK SECOND-FAMILY MEMBERS IN

When Frank's tagalong friend, Dan, came in, he sat down and almost immediately began discussing his own terrible problems. Dan lived with a single, alcoholic mother who brought different men back with her. Dan said he often stayed out all night because he was repulsed about going home. Frank seemed relieved that someone else besides him knew about Dan's bad situation. After seeing this small "family" of two for several weeks, I encouraged Dan, a chronic marijuana user himself, to come clean with his mother, or if he could not, to contact a drug program that would see him alone. *(Note: To find out whether or not you must advise parents before making any recommendations to a child's friend, check your state requirements.)*

As often happens, changes in one part of a system can have a pronounced ripple effect. When Dan entered a program and stopped using drugs, so did Frank; after Frank quit, so did his girlfriend. With these barriers down, Frank could become more honest with his parents, revealing to them how far into chaos his life had drifted.

Now more alert to second-family dynamics, when I began seeing Julia, a 14-year-old girl with bulimia, I asked her if she would like to invite her best friend, Laurie, to visit for a couple of meetings. She was glad to. *(Note: Whether you work in a clinic setting or privately, if you plan to see a second-family member for more than one or two meetings, it may be important to get the permission of the parents of your client by calling them. Check with agency guidelines. Discuss this with the teen in ongoing treatment and, if in your judgment it's necessary, call the parents, since they are responsible for payment.)* While Julia was withdrawn, secretive, and shy, Laurie was gregarious and talkative—a natural leader. Actually, however, Laurie was in more serious trouble than her friend. She had multiple sexual partners and was caught in the middle of a savage custody battle between her separating parents. It was obvious, too, that Julia was actually taking care of Laurie—acting as confidante, even receptacle, of Laurie's need to spill her guts.

Two weeks later, when Laurie's mask of bravado cracked, she asked if I could help her. After several phone calls to her parents emphasizing the truly perilous state of their daughter's situation (first, check on HIPAA privacy regulations), I persuaded them to enter divorce mediation rather than battling it out via lawyers. Once Laurie's parents had moderated their hostilities, she felt less frantic, and began attending a support group for girls with eating disorders. Because I had taken Laurie's problems seriously and freed Julia from the burden of saving her friend, Julia began to trust me more and started talking about her own difficulties with food and boys.

YOU MAY NEED PERMISSION
FROM THE SECOND-FAMILY LEADER

To cross rigid peer group boundaries, counselors often must get permission from an important second-family member. Sometimes the identity of the key peer group member is not immediately apparent. We are easily duped because (as discussed in Chapter 2) most media-obsessed kids are highly sophisticated users of pop psychology. Jared, for example, a 15-year-old with no connection of any importance to an adult, was ordered into drug counseling at his school. As is often the case, the counselor, Erica, thought everything was going well: Jared was polite and agreeable. Though he did not actually tell her much, she felt hopeful that once they "connected," he would open up—until he suddenly dropped therapy without warning or explanation.

Several months later, caught smoking marijuana, Jared was once more forced into counseling. At this point, Erica asked my advice, and I suggested she call his girlfriend, Jenny, treating her exactly as if she were a family member whose permission and cooperation were needed for counseling to continue. As the counselor soon found out, Jared and Jenny were absolute soulmates—mutual caretakers and protectors, best friends, lovers, quasi-siblings. Jenny had been deeply jealous of and anxious about Jared's first therapist; she could not tolerate an adult female's getting close to him.

But, on the second try, when Erica asked Jenny for her "permission" to see Jared, showing her the respect she needed, Jenny lost her defensiveness. Holding Jared's hand, she told Erica how Jared, who seemed exceptionally smooth and self-confident, was often so lonely at night that he could not sleep and turned to pot for relief. To help both cut down on pot smoking, Jenny said, she had taken to calling him every evening and talking until they dropped off with the phones in their hands.

Jared struggled for some time with his drug problem and long-ignored learning difficulties. But he accepted his parents' idea of random drug testing as a way to keep him on track—a major step for someone who had lived his life in secretiveness and hiding. Both he and Jenny were less isolated in the closed little world of each other's company; they talked more openly to their parents and began to experience themselves as individuals, separate from each other.

Friends Deepen the Relationship

FRIENDS SET A TONE OF OPENNESS

The presence of friends in the room loosens up the somewhat artificial teen–professional relationship. When an adolescent brings in friends, it helps her be open in ways that she might not normally be, if it's just the two of us talking.

Other kids, for one thing, make comments and observations she can't control. Welcoming friends in obviously conveys the message that I'm interested in all aspects of her life, including the kids she cares about. Jill, for example, often showed me snapshots of her pals. One day she appeared with two friends in person, and said, "I thought this would make them feel more real to you." Jill was right. The photos came to life. That meeting, and the exchanges we continued to have about school and about kids she knew, set the stage for Jill to feel comfortable bringing in, over time, just about every important friend. Jill was the first of many kids who by now volunteer to bring in photos of friends, and then the friends themselves. These kids are always energized when describing, in great detail, intimacies with those whom they want me to meet. Another brick in the wall of silence is removed.

OTHER PERSPECTIVES ENTER THE PICTURE

You gain new perspectives about your client, and this is immensely valuable. You already know what parents think, because you have been meeting with them. You know how a teen sees himself, which is also important. Yet many of the kids who come to treatment have major difficulties because they lack a broader perspective on who they are. To paraphrase Harry Stack Sullivan: We're psychologically healthy to the extent that we can see ourselves the way that other people see us. Friends add another dimension, and these different views eventually converge.

From a teen's friends, I get all kinds of impressions, including some that may be quite different from how my client presents himself. Jack, a boy I saw for some time, appeared to be a tough, macho kind of kid. Dressed head to toe in black, he was heavily into video games saturated with violence, acted supercool, and was pretty forbidding to the adults in his life. When several of his friends came to our session with him one day, however, these kids talked about Jack in totally different ways—somewhat to his embarrassment.

His friends mentioned all the times in which Jack was a caretaker. He stayed on the phone for hours when a friend's father died after a long illness; he went out of his way to be with someone who was having trouble with another close friend; he came up with remarkably thoughtful presents for others. None of this had come out in the talking he and I did together, until his second family contributed different perspectives on who he was. That other side of Jack became not only part of our conversation, but part of my ability to more fully understand him.

FRIENDS CAN TURN OUT TO BE YOUR CONSULTANTS

The second family often fills in pieces that I myself may not really understand. One boy, Paul, for example, brought a friend to his session, a girl he'd known since elementary school. I was able to ask her why, in her opinion, Paul had such a hard time studying. Her response was revealing: She thought that his parents weren't strict enough, that they gave in too much, and that he never developed the skill of studying. He simply had not learned to buckle down and get to it. This she saw as a family problem as much as a Paul problem. After explaining her perspective to me, she turned to him and said: "You know Paul, I really think you'd be a lot better off if you could start trying and doing some of the work. Things wouldn't be so hard for you if you just got into the habit of trying."

That kind of help was unexpected; it arose naturally out of the discussion. She was right. Paul's parents were seriously divided as to how much they should demand of Paul, and he was falling through the cracks into academic oblivion.

FRIENDS WILL TELL YOUR CLIENT WHAT'S WORRYING THEM

When you bring in an adolescent's friends, you may hear them express strong opinions, delivered in a tactful manner. Teens seem to naturally use a relational–behavioral approach. It is wrong to view the peer group as only a source of trouble, as we so often are encouraged to do. Kids look out for each other; with certain safeguards, they will speak up when someone is going over the line or drifting into potential danger. More than once I've heard a client's friend say to him, point-blank: "I think you're smoking dope too much. I can't stop you, it's not my thing, please don't think I'm laying this on you. But that's what I think." It is almost always done with a degree of humility and graciousness.

Alex, a gay adolescent, came in with his boyfriend, Carl. Carl, who had many problems himself, at one point turned to Alex and said: "You're always worrying about my issues, because they're sort of dramatic. But I worry about how harsh you are toward yourself." Looking at me, Carl said, "Can you help him with that? Because he's always helping me instead of taking care of himself."

A 13-year-old girl and two of her friends spent some of the session bantering back and forth and gossiping about boys and so on. Then one remarked, "You know, Kaliyah, you're very moody, and your moods are really hard for all of us to take, even though we really love you. I hope you talk to the doctor about your moodiness."

Opinions like these are invaluable—delivered not from an adult, not as a lecture, but in an empathically firm way from friend to friend. When such moments happen, they can begin a dialogue about some of the more difficult things kids are into that they don't want to talk about themselves.

FRIENDS ARE SOURCES OF INVALUABLE INFORMATION

Opening the door to friends is especially important during dangerous times, when you are moving past gray-zone behavior, starting to worry deeply about the adolescent you're seeing.

A 15-year-old girl, Brenda, was becoming self-destructive. She had not triggered a loss of confidentiality yet, but was on her way. Brenda acted out by drinking too much, not remembering where she was, and ending up with kids she didn't know. Two friends in her second family alerted me to these behaviors and said to me, with her there, "We're really worried about Brenda, because we think she's in bad shape right now and she could hurt herself. Somebody should know."

In another case I was supervising, friends told the therapist they were worried about his client because she was making herself throw up every day. Typical of girls in this culture, they had tolerance for all varieties of eating difficulties. But they sensed their friend was in deeper-than-usual trouble, because she could not stop herself from vomiting at least once a day. They wanted to tell *some* adult that this was going on, since her parents didn't suspect a thing.

In a poignant meeting I had with my patient and his girlfriend, high school sweethearts who had been involved for years, I listened to them—like an old married couple—bicker back and forth. Then, in the roller-coaster style of adolescence, they'd turn affectionate and cozy with each other. Toward the end of the session, she suddenly said to him, "You know, you scare the shit out of me with your driving. I'm really frightened about how fast you go. Have you told Ron about what you do?" He hadn't. This was a good kid with (as my 13-year-old son, Sam, would say) an "Achilles-tendency": He loved speed. In fact, he had secretly amassed dozens of motor vehicle tickets, for parking violations and minor infractions, concrete indicators something dangerous was brewing that I had no knowledge of. Almost incidentally, then, I learned about the risks my client was taking every day—a detail that led to heated debates with me and, eventually, a focused family session.

In each case, having friends in the session allowed me to gain access to information about a teen who was in dangerous territory, and to then be able to address the issue with the child directly or with his parents.

FRIENDS HELP YOU GRASP THE ETHOS OF YOUR CLIENT'S GROUP

Meeting with friends allows you to learn about the ambience of the second family, what the rules and expectations are. This is just as important as finding out the ethos of the first family at home. Damien often appeared with a bunch of friends. Armed with all the paraphernalia of "slackers"—skateboards, in-line roller-blades, hip-hop banter, and cool gesticulations—I quickly sensed (though most 12-year-olds would have realized it immediately), this group was one that smoked a lot of pot. If I had not met everyone and gotten such a clear message, I'm not sure I would have grasped the degree of smoking Damien took for granted in his daily life. Meeting his friends sped up our work in a significant way.

Over time I met the friends of 14-year-old Charlotte. She partied famously on weekends, but was moody and highly argumentative during the week. I saw that each of her girlfriends was more of a drama queen than the next. After just one meeting I could well understand why Charlotte considered her own precipitous changes in mood to be the norm, rather than a sign of any pain or suffering.

Another client was a boy who did not try very hard in school; he spent most of his time practicing "extreme" sports—skateboarding, snowboarding, and the like. Although he suffered from a clear learning difficulty, he had developed a reputation among the adults in his life as a lazy and indifferent kid. Over time, as I met his friends, I began to realize that these kids were incredibly kind and caretaking toward each other. There were never any insults about poor grades, never any put-downs. The ethos of the group seemed to be that everyone should look out for each other. School was secondary; nurturance and bonding were what really mattered. To master his learning issue meant jeopardizing his unbelievably comfortable niche—an invaluable understanding for our work.

In contrast, another group of boys I met were passionately misogynistic. Girls were literally referred to as "chickenheads," people who had no thoughts, only bodies and who should be treated in the most demeaning ways possible. It was revealing (and discouraging) to understand how antifemale this postfeminist group of 21st-century boys were. It took years for the group's "fraternity of contempt" to settle down, finally dissipating when one of its leaders broke ranks and actually fell in love with a girl.

MEETING FRIENDS HELPS YOU UNDERSTAND THE DEGREE OF PEER PRESSURE

Typically, as kids move along a developmental continuum, the intensity of peer pressure actually decreases. While there may be terrible pressure during younger adolescence, as kids get older they ease into a more tolerant, live-and-let live attitude. Allowances are made for individual differences. Within some groups, however, peer pressure continues to be intense, whatever the age. This is critical to know. Meeting friends helps you understand it.

Cole, a boy I was seeing because of nonstop fighting with his parents and stepparents, was secretly part of a group in which there was tremendous pressure to vandalize property and write graffiti. To this urban posse, desecration of property was their route to "celebrity." No matter what time of night, no matter how dangerous the assignment, Cole could *never* turn these militant kids down. Forays onto others' turf or rewriting other kids' signatures was an invitation to brutal fights and plots for revenge. Peer pressure within this particular second family only diminished when several members were arrested and spent two harrowing days in a prison holding cell.

One 14-year-old girl, Cathy, belonged to a group organized around beauty and cruelty. They were "queen bees" who intimidated everybody, including each other. Meeting a couple of those kids helped me understand how they *had* to maintain a certain look and hard-ass attitude that established their dominance. Cathy's mother was incensed and humiliated. She had grown up in the South, believing in civility and compassionate values. To her, this overt cruelty was a deep personal affront, an attack against everything she held dear. But the glamour of the group was far more than Cathy could resist. Her mother's meetings with me were filled with ineffective complaints. My work with Cathy never gained enough traction to break the group's hold on her values. It was only when she moved on to another school and found a more diverse second family that Cathy began to change.

Some groups, on the other hand, allow each other *a lot of latitude*. In another second family that frequently smoked dope, there was absolutely *no* pressure to do so. Over time, many of the kids stopped smoking, and nobody tried to pull them back into it. This particular group prided itself on a live-and-let-live ethos, making the work with my client far less complicated. When he began buckling down in school I sensed no disdain from his buddies. As I observed for years, each child went his or her own way. They stayed fast friends, but moved along their individual paths, without needing to "be the same."

FRIENDS HELP YOU LEARN ABOUT THE BIG-PICTURE WORLD OF TEENS

A lot of what I have learned about the new adolescence has come not only from clients, but from their friends. Sitting with three or four kids amounts to having a focus group in the room. Being together seems to encourage a kind of assertiveness that teens enjoy amongst their peers, but rarely with adults. I ask opinions about all kinds of issues, and I will hear what they think, with little censoring: about drinking, how rock concerts can be dangerous, or the way my client's parents are viewed by other kids. They will tell me how clueless they feel parents are in general, what authority parents should have, what they really need from adults. Kids frankly discuss their ever-changing definitions of substances, sex, cheating, and dating practices.

To check out what I hear, every couple of years I measure these group responses against large-scale national studies on teen trends such as the Center for Disease Control statistics on mental illness, Youth and High-Risk data, The Kaiser Family Foundation surveys, Planned Parenthood research, and the CASA (National Center on Addiction and Substance Abuse at Columbia University) database, to name just a few sources. It has astonished me how accurate the interviews with my clients' friends have been on every one of these subjects.

In fact, most of what we hear by inviting friends in is several years ahead of formal surveys. For example, national researchers are beginning to recognize that old definitions of high school sex may be changing for kids—what was once reserved for *after* intercourse is now happening *before,* rewriting the meaning of "abstinence" and active sexuality. Researchers are just now spotting trends that I'd heard for years in my workshops and my consulting room. Meeting with kids in groups to talk about "ordinary life" keeps profession-

---

Getting Smarter with Age: Some of What I've Learned about Teen Life—from Friends of Clients

◆ The secret world of loft parties and raves.

◆ The gradual increase in binge drinking.

◆ Peer pressure in younger, elementary school kids.

◆ The new anxiety and increased childhood stress.

◆ The trend that girls are catching up to boys in high-risk behaviors.

◆ What kids respect in parents today—what teens need from adults.

◆ The increase of casual anger and revenge between peers.

◆ Current redefinitions of sex.

◆ The increase of nonsexual friendship between boys and girls.

◆ The intensity of homophobia in middle school boys.

◆ The reality that consequences count as much as emotional intelligence.

◆ That middle school and college are the fastest growing high-risk periods.

◆ How often siblings introduce brothers and sisters to substance use.

---

als up-to-date about subtle changes in the way teens think and live. No clinician should ignore what the kids are saying.

BRING IN THE SIBLINGS, TOO

Because we have two kids in our own family, I think of an older sibling as being a protective presence in a younger sibling's life. It was sobering to learn a different truth when I invited siblings into meetings (without parents). From one after another, *I learned that kids are often introduced to high-risk behaviors by an older brother or sister.* It was an older sibling who got a client drunk, or allowed a younger sib to hang out with the group and to witness (or become involved with) sexual acting out. All of this is, of course, hidden from parents. The older sibling invariably doesn't feel that he or she is doing something wrong. Just the opposite. As one high school senior said to me, "I'd rather have my kid brother get trashed with me than with a stranger. I'll teach him the ropes instead of having him learn in a dangerous way."

Over time, then, I discovered the wisdom of arranging "sibling sessions" whenever I can. Siblings have a profound understanding about pressures at home, and often know the friends of the child I'm seeing much better than parents do. In addition, an older sib can be a potential ally, because he or she has passed through this territory before. They can speak from personal experience about living more safely, even as they introduce a younger brother or sister to second-family realities.

In a session with 15-year-old Owen and his college-age older sister, Erin, she talked about her extensive experimentation with drugs, how deeply into that world she got, and how she finally pulled herself out. Erin was concerned that Owen might have an addictive personality. She saw some of that in herself and in their parents. During the session, she talked forcefully to Owen, and clearly a lot of this was news to him. She made a powerful impact on Owen's views about alcohol, his substance of choice. While Erin's comments didn't stop Owen from drinking, she helped me gain some footing in my efforts to slow him down.

Mariel, a 14-year-old client, had a 10-year-old sister, Paula, whom I asked in for a session. From the way the two talked, I saw firsthand how viciously they tormented each other—using words like "fat" and "stupid," zeroing in on exactly what each most feared or disliked about herself. But Paula, the younger sister, was the one who really spilled the beans about the dynamics of taunting that went on at home. In our "siblings only" meeting, Paula described the subtle provocations she inflicted on her sister—breathing on her, speaking in a squeaky voice that she knew would drive Mariel crazy, and so on. In these ways, Paula very effectively got her big sister in trouble with their mom and stepdad. Mariel always seemed to be exploding in anger, and couldn't help but be viewed as "the problem." Their parents had a set perception of the two girls that did not accurately reflect what was really going on—the subterranean territory that exists in the world of siblings, far away from busy parents.

When I met Olivia, the older sister of 12-year-old Maggie, I could see there was no way Maggie could feel good about herself. A girl with learning difficulties to start with, she happened to be part of a family that included a very accomplished mother and sister. Olivia was one of the quickest, most charismatic kids I'd ever met. Maggie didn't stand a chance against her. Meeting Olivia with Maggie opened my eyes, allowing us to talk from shared experience about what it must be like to live in a family with a sister who was an absolute star.

Parent to Parent

You've just met with your client and a group of his friends. You learn that one of the other kids is being treated badly at home, or is thinking of running away. In openly dangerous situations such as these, you may decide (if you have time, first checking with your agency on ethics or privacy regulations) to work with your client's parents to determine if, when, and how they might talk to the parents of the friend.

Twelve-year-old Sean was verbally abused by Alec, one of his so-called best friends. Sean's parents knew Alec; they believed he was a fine friend for their son. They had no idea of the boy's sadistic behavior, because Alec was a great actor and his attacks were always conducted out of earshot. After this was revealed during a session I had with Sean and another of his friends, Sean's parents and I discussed ways they could bring up the matter with Alec's parents. After practicing, they figured out how to approach his mother and father, and how to talk about what was happening in a way that might not make them too defensive.

Fourteen-year-old Erica brought three friends to a session one day, and in the course of our talk they mentioned that another girl they knew had serious issues around eating. Interestingly, this candor during the session somehow encouraged Erica to open up more with her mother. That night, she brought up with Mom that one of her friends was in real trouble—eating strangely (saying after a small bowl of soup: "I'm full"), compulsively exercising, talking endlessly about food. Erica and her mother worked out a way Mom could approach that girl's mother, to at least bring up their concerns.

It is great when a relationship duo come in. The pair will usually talk openly to me—and to each other—about aspects of their relationship, I'm then able to relay some of that information to the parents of my client. Very often one or both sets of parents have a hard time accepting this adolescent romance, or they simply don't know much about it at all. What can happen next—and I've seen this more than once—*is that the two sets of parents start talking to each other for the first time.* They create an alliance that helps them become far more effective regarding many ordinary, but worrisome, issues.

With my encouragement, Lauren's mother finally called up Mark's mother. The two kids had been passionately in love for months, but their parents had never even spoken. One phone call started regular conversations between the two moms. They discussed how late the kids were staying out, whether or not they were getting enough sleep, why they had to be on the phone until 3:00 A.M., and how much "freedom" both mothers wanted to give the young couple. After creating some ground rules and accepting this relationship was "the real deal," Lauren's mother invited Mark to go on a vacation with the family. Parent talking to parent created tolerance for an adolescent relationship that had been previously driven underground.

However, parent talking to parent doesn't always work. After a session with 14-year-old Michael and a couple of his friends, I felt it was necessary to let Michael's mother know that the group was regularly getting together to drink in another boy's empty house. Michael's mother immediately (against my advice), called up one of the other parents and said, "Do you know our kids are drinking six-packs in this kid's basement every weekend? We've got to do something." She was right; it *was* dangerous behavior, and they *did* have to do something. But she handled the issue impulsively, without planning or careful thought. The outcome was disastrous for

Michael: He was ostracized by his group for the better part of a year—the scariest consequence of all for a teen. Somewhere in the middle of that awful time, Michael's mom said to me, "It wasn't worth it. I shouldn't have done what I did, in the way I did it."

*   *   *

Fortunately, bringing in a teen's friends usually has a more positive outcome: As the working relationship opens up, an atmosphere of listening migrates to the first family at home. Over and over I have seen that as greater openness develops among a child, her friends, and me, the more I am able to help parents achieve the same. They invite their kid's friends to the house more often; they see what actually goes on in the second family. Occasionally, as parents get to know a child's friend better, they become worried about her and work hard to get her parents to accept the idea of counseling, sometimes using me as a conduit.

Invariably, I see how most parents can stretch beyond rigid patterns or cluelessness and become more realistic about the strengths as well as the weaknesses of their child's peer group. That knowledge, of course, allows for greater connection with their once-distant teen. Ultimately it allows parents to more intelligently guide what is going on in an adolescent's tumultuous life.

*   *   *

If "It takes a village . . . ," it may be time to include some of its most colorful and troublesome, yet invaluable citizens over to "your house." You will never be the same. After this door is opened and you have welcomed the second family in, you start to think younger.

THE REAL IN RELATIONAL

Challenging Ourselves
to Stay Three-Dimensional with Teens

> For all the reasons described in these pages, 21st-century kids suffer from not experiencing enough genuine adult presence. In order to break through to teens we must feel real to them, or we are wasting everyone's time.

We have come full circle, back to the edge of relatedness. All the clinical techniques in the world aren't worth a damn if we don't feel real to the kids we try to help. Staying three-dimensional is not so easy for us therapists, though.

Long after my inspiring experience as a camp counselor, the early years of professional training seemed to squeeze some of the life out of me in the consulting room. Mental health professionals, after all, spend a lot of time learning how *not* to be real in the room. Controversy over how we ought to be spans the century from Freud to the new millennium. Regardless of orientation, most of us are, at least in theory (i.e., the way we report our work in training or supervision), the slightly removed professional—one part technical directive, one part clinical observation, and one part measured tone. Unfortunately, we don't always realize how this two-dimensionality *recreates* a major problem for teens in a postmodern world.

When kids were being squashed by an authoritarian culture, it made sense to ensure enough emotional space for young clients to develop a separate sense of self. The world has obviously changed over the past two decades. I've asked hundreds of kids, *What adult has made a real difference in your life?* By and large, a theme emerges: The best therapists or counselors they had seen, the best teachers, the most effective parents at home were those who came across with *clarity and emotion*. Kids could actually hear these adults. They stood out from the brash and noisy culture all around. Teens and preteens describe grown-ups who are *really there*.

A 12-year-old boy said about his sixth-grade teacher: "Yeah, she'd lose it sometimes. But, she was for real. We knew she meant what she said."

A 15-year-old girl said: "I went to a lot of shrinks, but this one was different. When she said something, she was out there and I'd pay attention."

A 16-year-old junior remembered his drama teacher from middle school: "That guy said things clear as a bell, he was so emotional—I even remember some of what he taught me."

Other kids, unfortunately, have had very different experiences. In one way or another they describe adults as two-dimensional figures who are afraid to make their presence felt. Many have specifically said about mental health professionals: "What's with you therapists? Who told you to be like this? You're so boring and phony it's unbelievable. How do you expect kids to talk or listen to you?"

Personal engagement, the relational "edge" to use Darlene Ehrenberg's term, is *the* quality that teens point to. Kids need somebody real. It makes total sense in today's world.

Raised on Special Effects and Reality TV

Children are raised on special effects and stark reality in every possible medium—network and cable television, reality shows, DVDs, video games, advertisements, magazines, and, every night, online. They are accustomed to drama and melodrama, instant action and interaction, intense stimulation and everyday special effects. Contrast this larger-than-life reality to the fact that almost every teen-ager has secondhand therapy experience. Endless "How did that make you feel?" media scenes became such a slow-moving cliché that edgy "challenge and change" formats took over. Kids like it raw, and the word on the street is that most of us child profession-als are boring! For teens, "Dr. Phil" is the real deal. Oprah still rocks. Simon tells it like it is.

"I'M READY FOR MY CLOSE-UP, MR. DE MILLE"

A lack of therapeutic flair is not only inconsistent with digitally en-hanced drama, it doesn't even match the flair of ordinary adoles-cence. Adolescents are consummate aficionados of the juicy close-up shot. They are able to turn the most mundane event into gut-wrenching dish.

Debbie, the mother of 15-year-old Suzanne, greeted her daughter one afternoon: "Hi, sweetie. How'd it go today?" Su-zanne had gone to meet a friend at the mall, no big deal—just an-other day. Mom expected to hear little of substance. Then Suzanne started to tell her tale of woe: She and Molly were to meet Megan at a store in the mall. But Megan didn't show up. Suzanne and Molly started to argue: Should they call her? Should they leave? They also tried on a whole bunch of sweaters and jeans while they were debating about what to do with Megan. The impatient store manager was an "incredible tight-ass" and tried to get rid of them. Finally, they decided to leave a note for Megan with a nicer (young) salesperson there, explaining where they were going. Megan showed up after they left, but the store-kid didn't pass along the note, and Megan thought she'd been ditched. Mean-while, Suzanne and Molly had called Emma and met up with *her* in another part of the mall. Still another friend saw Suzanne, Molly, and Emma. She then bumped into Megan and told her about the other three. Megan was furious, Molly and Suzanne learned later. But by that time they had gotten a ride to Megan's house and asked her mom, Diane, if she knew where Megan was. Now Diane flew into a rage, because Megan had been told not to go shopping at all, since she was supposed to come straight home to babysit. Suzanne and Molly felt really, really upset, not only because they had ditched Megan—although they actually hadn't—but because it was the store manager's fault for bothering the kid so much that he probably forgot their message. Now Megan's mother was furious with her daughter. And it wasn't totally their fault for ratting out Megan to her mother—"Right, Mom?"

Recounting this story to me, Debbie added, "All I said was, 'How was your day?' " Like any teen, her daughter was capable of turning a Seinfeldian afternoon about "absolutely nothing" into Shakespearean high drama.

A more serious example: Richard and Emily exchanged a series of e-mails, which Richard showed one of my supervisees during a session. Emily was mad because she thought of Richard as a boyfriend, but he actually liked a friend of hers. So, Emily sent Richard an e-mail saying that she had just seen the list of finalists in a statewide science competition, and he wasn't on it. Richard freaked out, and wrote a furious e-mail back to Emily, who replied that she was going to cut herself if he didn't stop going out with her friend. Richard was now even more upset, but mainly kept talking about how he failed to make it in the science competition. Emily wrote back accusing him of being incredibly selfish—all he cared about was the stupid award—and couldn't he see that she was really hurting? He wrote back asking how she could be so callous when his life's dream had just gone down the toilet. Now Emily wrote back admitting that she'd made up the entire business about the finalist's list, just so he could know firsthand the feeling of rejection that she experienced because he liked her friend.

"I HATE BEING BORED!"

One final ingredient in the developmental stew of contemporary adolescence is an allergic reaction to boredom—which roughly translated means moments without being able to multitask. Picture an ordinary evening—a kid on the computer "doing homework," listening to CDs he's burned off the Internet, instant-messaging five friends at the same time, while on the phone with two "call waiting" conversations, TV droning in the background, and playing online poker to fill in those barren seconds of down-time. Now, ask yourself: Is it possible to capture a teen's attention with therapeutic phrases like *"That must really have been upsetting to you?"* Will most adolescents even register such a hackneyed state-ment, let alone focus sufficiently to discuss the important deci-sions that must be made everyday in their lives?

Toward a Three-Dimensional Therapist

During the last decade, the relational model and self psychology's "intersubjectivity" have been widely discussed in the treatment of adults. According to these perspectives, "therapeutic action" oc-curs in the exchange created by two *real* people in the consulting room. Over time, each comes to more clearly understand their ex-perience and impact on the other. The two-dimensional therapist is being replaced by a more complex, human therapist. *This relation-al thinking has not fully impacted the world of treating teens.* Given the nature of 21st-century adolescence, this is a shame. For all the rea-sons described in these pages, kids suffer from *not* experiencing enough genuine adult presence. In order to break through to teens we must feel real to them or we are wasting everyone's time. We need a frame that allows us our humanity and provides guidelines for staying three-dimensional in the work.

SAY IT WITH FEELING—OR DON'T SAY IT AT ALL

In previous chapters I have described countless ordinary yet hair-raising experiences adolescents discuss. I have heard most of these examples not once, but dozens of times in various permutations. Peter is planning a date in an abandoned garage with a complete stranger he met in cyberspace. Ten-year-old Theo is teased relent-lessly by other kids for being "gay." Erica is mercilessly demeaned by classmates because her mother died. Shawna talks about oral sex with a bunch of boys at "rainbow parties"—where boys paint lip-gloss on their penises and the "winner" is the girl who ends up with the most color on her lips. Lewis regularly smokes pot in the bathroom at his middle school. Anna is threatened online not to come to school if she wants to live. Mary and Herbert write graffiti on abandoned buildings 10 stories high. A bunch of high school boys and girls line up strippers for an afternoon of lap dancing in a neighbor's home.

The list is endless.

Working with teens, we hear these stories all the time. It is impossible not to react without a full range of feeling: outrage, sadness, shock, fear, excitement, envy, relief, and so on. To stay three-dimensional and to be heard, you must *respond* in some honest way that reflects your internal experience—in your own style, in your own words—in a way your client absolutely cannot miss. "How do you feel about what's happening?" is static in a multi-gigahertz, high-tech world.

When Peter first told me about his online dating scheme, I said: "Are you out of your mind?" To Erica, who was tormented about her mother: "I feel like I want to *cry* when I hear what those girls *did to you*." To Lewis, who smoked up in middle school: "Are you trying to drive me insane?" To Ernie, who talked about really liking a girl, and how every adult told him high school relationships are doomed, I said: *"With all my heart,* I believe there's a chance for you and Chloe to make it. *It is possible,"* I almost whispered.

The words are not unusual, but we often flatten our feelings because we consider them unprofessional or nontherapeutic. Yet in every one of these situations, kids saw me with different eyes. Their expressions said, "Here's somebody who gets what I'm saying, and who cares about me. Maybe I'll even listen."

UNDERSCORE WHAT YOU SAY IN PHYSICAL WAYS

Actions, not just words, add drama and authenticity to the moment. Years ago at my agency, I watched from behind a one-way mirror a family session that left a lasting impression. An adolescent started talking about himself in derogatory ways. The therapist nearly jumped out of her seat and shouted at the boy, "Don't you ever say anything so negative about yourself again! Never!" I was taken aback—a therapist should not do this, I thought. But, obviously this teen client thought differently. He brightened up and opened up—about what life was really like behind *his* wall of silence.

Almost a decade ago, I worked with a withdrawn, young adolescent girl, Lisa, who mumbled the very few words she chose to say. Failing in school, Lisa was diagnosed as ADD, oppositional, and selectively mute. Finally, I suggested to Lisa that she walk around the room a bit, just to settle in. I thought maybe our stuck psychical positions might be loosened by a physical change. Lisa liked the idea, and I trailed her with my notebook. Lisa mumbled; I yelled, "What? What did you say?" I'd ask Lisa to repeat herself, so I could take notes. The more I walked and wrote behind her, the more she began to laugh and yell back at me, talking in a way that could actually be understood. Lisa's shyness reflected her quiet position in both her stepfamily at home and her second family of friends. Along with attentional issues, Lisa's withdrawn quality was intensified by an undiagnosed language-processing problem.

Another girl, Tina, 15, described to me how she had gotten drunk over the weekend, stole a car, and took off for a wild, high-speed joyride. Sitting in my "official" therapist recliner, I moved the seat back as far as it could go, so I was almost parallel to the floor. I looked at her and said, "I feel totally flattened, like a pancake. I can't believe you took that chance with your life and everybody else's. I'm stunned." Demonstrating physically how squashed I felt snapped Tina out of her trance. She was able to see, at least for a moment, that this episode might be something important. There were no miracles. My reaction created just a *slight* awareness about her downwardly spiraling life.

Thirteen-year-old Willie is one of the boys with whom I throw a ball back and forth. Willie often made remarks that were provocative and insulting to me. These casual put-downs were similar to the way he spoke to everybody else in his life. I said, "I don't like the way you're insulting me. If I were a kid, I'd go out of my way to make trouble for you." To underline my feelings, I'd throw the ball back much harder—not hard enough to hurt, but hard enough to let him know I was angry and he better pay attention to his impact on me.

At times I've walked out of the consulting room. When Brian told me, with a grin on his face, about prank-calling older people dozens of times, I said: "Brian, what you're doing is outrageous. You seem unable to think about the effect you're having on these people. You know what, I have to take a break from you for a minute." When I returned (a minute later), Brian was willing to talk about what he was doing. It was no different than the childishly annoying way he often treated his parents and friends—one of the reasons he so frequently got into fights.

Body language matters to teens, as it does to everyone. A challenging relationship ought not to be dependent only on the spoken word or a well-modulated tone. You don't want to be a prisoner, stuck on your own clinical throne.

IT'S ALL RELATIVE: CHANGING SESSION LENGTH
TO MIRROR SESSION CONTENT

Another action that often gets through is changing the parameters of treatment. As long as we fill out insurance and agency forms accurately, charge less, or make up lost time, there is nothing sacrosanct about "the treatment hour." Especially with teens, flexibility sends a message kids hear. So, there are times I will cut the session short or lengthen it because I want to make sure just one point actually gets through.

For example, Aiden, a 16-year-old, was stuck on the notion that his girlfriend *had* to give him oral sex. If she didn't, it meant she didn't really care about him. More important, he was not getting what he thought every other guy was getting, casually or from girlfriends. "If she's not going to give me head, I'll break up with her!" Aiden (and increasing numbers of other boys during the past five years) simply couldn't get past this thought. I let him know that although I understood where this was coming from, his wish was the exact opposite of what was involved in becoming a man. I wanted one message to get through from our discussion: for Aiden to agree to go for an entire weekend without turning the oral sex issue into a huge fight between him and this girl he really liked. After we negotiated thoroughly about his weekend goal, Aiden finally relented and agreed. I stopped the session at that exact moment. I didn't want this hard-fought agreement to be buried by the next dramatic issue that was sure to come up. Instead, I scheduled a 15-minute session before the weekend to see what he was feeling, and to underline its importance once more. Aiden actually remembered our discussion—in the meantime he'd asked none other than his father about what to do. Dad gave it his full attention and "sensitively" said, "Hey, there's more to life than getting head."

Melissa, who had endless arguments every weekend with her parents over homework, talked about her "bizarre" parents, about how they never left her alone. In fact, Melissa was pestering *them* all the time for help, then blowing a fuse when they didn't do it right—which prompted their intense reactions. When we finally began approaching *her part* in this awful interaction, Melissa became stubborn and annoyed with me. This dance between us seemed stuck (just as it was at home), so I temporarily ended it by saying, "Let's take a break here. In a few minutes we'll go over it again. My head is spinning." Continuing to take breaks, Melissa and I short-circuited our cycle of frustration and anger. The meeting went over about 15 minutes. By the end of it, though, Melissa got a tiny glimpse into her contribution. We had inadvertently stumbled onto a better format of working collaboratively: Don't plow ahead, and build in "time outs" to cool down.

CREATE AN ENACTMENT BETWEEN YOU AND YOUR CLIENT

Structural family therapy's "enactment" is a useful tool not just in family meetings, but in individual sessions with adolescents. A spirited dialogue between you and your client almost always turns in to a mirror-image reflection of what is actually happening at home or in the second family. Once the interaction gets going, your message—insight, self-awareness, and a plan of action—can be absorbed in a genuine, experiential way. Because the exchange is relationally true, it cuts through the distracting noise that consistently diffuses adolescent attention in the room.

The enactment is not about "venting." It needs a particular focus or a specific point you're trying to convey. With 16-year-old Mike, the aim of the enactment was to help him develop greater empathy—a quality he sorely lacked with his parents and his friends, an expression of a nonverbal learning disability that got him into trouble every day. Mike's graduation from middle school was coming up, and he wanted the celebration to be held in his home. Mike's reasons were logical: the party should be fun, no pressure, just a relaxed time. His mother agreed at first, but as the day got closer and the guest list grew longer, she started "freaking out" about having so many people in her small house. She felt she couldn't handle it, and began talking about renting a cheap space in a nearby community center.

Mike was furious, displaying anger without empathy—the issue that got him to me in the first place. He came to our meeting visibly upset with his mom. I listened to his gripes for a while. Then he and I had the following exchange:

THERAPIST: You won't like what I'm going to tell you, but I don't agree with you about this.

MIKE: Why not?

THERAPIST: Because, look, I like you, but I think I understand your mom not wanting to have this party at home.

MIKE: It's unfair!

THERAPIST: I don't expect you to agree. I just want you to hear my side and try to understand it.

MIKE: What about my side? *You're* not getting it.

THERAPIST: I heard it. I *am* on your side, too. You want to have fun. You want it to be easy and you think your mother is being unfair. But, it's important to empathize with me anyway. At least try to get why I think hundreds of people in the house may be freaking her out.

We went back and forth. Mike began shouting about the unfairness of it all.

MIKE: You don't understand what I'm talking about.

THERAPIST: (*with intensity*) I do. I was so self-conscious about how I looked, I didn't want pictures at my graduation. But I lost that one, just like you're going to lose on this one.

MIKE: That's totally different. You can rip up pictures afterwards. I'll have these memories my whole life.

THERAPIST: Look, I want you to try to see it from my perspective, what it felt like for me.

Around and around we went for the entire session, an enactment specifically focused on empathy. We parted with this discussion still in full blast. A couple of days later, I received a call from Mike's mother. "I don't know what you did," she said, "but it was the first time that Mike let me explain how frightened I was, that I just couldn't handle this party. He didn't agree to it, but at least he tried to hear me." That was the result I had hoped the enactment might create.

*   *   *

Fifteen-year-old Patsy was an adolescent I worked with in a neighborhood agency. As you will immediately see, Patsy created "enactments" wherever she went, making those around her deeply uncomfortable. Some background: At the beginning of our work, I told Patsy she could talk to me about anything, and say whatever she wanted. Here's how the dialogue went:

PATSY: So, how big is your dick?

THERAPIST: What?

PATSY: You heard me. You said I could say anything.

THERAPIST: Whatever I said, forget it. I won't answer that.

PATSY: You're hiding something.

THERAPIST: Listen, the most important thing is how astonishingly uncomfortable I feel. That's not what I meant when I said you could ask me whatever, and I think you know that. What are you doing?

PATSY: Nothing. I just always say what's on my mind.

THERAPIST: All the time?

PATSY: Pretty much.

THERAPIST: And this gets you what you want from people?

PATSY: They're not going to like me anyway, so I'll just have some fun, with them.

THERAPIST: Well, you're right. At this moment, I don't like you at all. (*long pause, with Patsy saying nothing*) Because what you said was unnecessarily provocative.

PATSY: Well, I'm not gonna change. I like being unpredictable.

THERAPIST: No matter how it makes someone else feel? No matter how it made me feel, just then?

PATSY: Listen, do you think it's different in my world? Do you think they treat me any way except like a piece of ass? This is my world, and if you want to understand me, you just better get used to it.

THERAPIST: Part of what happens here in this room is that you understand me, too, my world, too. It's not just about your feelings. It's never just about your feelings. Mine count also.

Patsy's approach to other people backfired in terms of being able to really get what she wanted. Our enactment in the room momentarily helped Patsy see her impact and hear another's experience in a safe way.

Transformations

The most important barometer of what is going on behind a teen's wall of silence are the signals your client triggers in *you*! In all therapy situations there are countertransferential responses we either chalk up to our own bits of "craziness" or label as "unprofessional." But gut responses are uncannily precise guideposts to unaddressed issues—issues kids have not been discussing or are glibly lying about, or ones representative of hidden family dynamics.

This is particularly true with adolescents. Their death-defying behavior, their harsh views on life, the raw way they speak inevitably provoke countertransference in the relationship. Adolescents (like adults with borderline and bipolar diagnoses or active addiction disorders) set off extreme reactions in professionals. Unfortunately, we berate ourselves for unacceptable experiences and tend to maintain a set of "double books" when we report to peers or supervisors about our emotions with young clients. In recent years, however, this view is changing. The writings of interpersonal-relational psychologists Irwin Hoffman (1983), and especially Edgar A. Levenson (1972) have helped therapists understand that feelings patients provoke should not be reflexively dismissed or considered shameful. They are signals to be addressed.

In 1972, psychoanalyst Edgar A. Levenson wrote *The Fallacy of Understanding*. In this book, and many subsequent articles that have had a profound impact on the world of relational psychoanalysis, Levenson describes how therapists cannot help repeating aspects of a patient's unresolved family relationships. So, for example, despite our best intentions with a client whose mother has been neglectful or harsh, we find ourselves at times acting inexplicably inattentive or indifferent. The unconscious pull exerted by a patient to "transform" (Levenson's word) his or her therapist into acting out underlying family dynamics is so compelling that no amount of safeguarding can entirely prevent it. Nor should it.

Levenson does not regard this transformation of the therapist as an evil to be sidestepped whenever possible but, rather, as an unsurpassed therapeutic tool. Recognizing how we've been transformed can cast a here-and-now spotlight on the often elusive beliefs that sustain a person's worldview and his or her approach to a problem. Pulling ourselves out of these transformations can be some of the crucial moments in our work, offering new strategies for kids as well as mothers and fathers.

When I first applied Levenson's idea of transformation to interventions with families, it was almost shocking how relevant it was. First, transformations happen immediately—sometimes within the first phone contact. For example, on the phone, setting up an initial meeting, I found myself acting extremely hassled and curt toward a mother. Later, I found out Mom's chief complaint was how rude and frenzied her daughter acted toward *her*! Second, the *way* we are transformed is a vital diagnostic indicator that helps us sift through the enormous amount of information families throw our way. Third, in order to make use of this information, we need to look carefully at our own experience during exchanges with kids and parents and how we act on that experience. For most helping professionals, however, this is easier said than done.

Many of us who work with children and families were never taught to think relationally, to keep alive a running internal dialogue along the lines of "What do I feel now?" or "Is this experience unusual for me?" or "Am I acting in a way that expresses these feelings?"—in short, "How am I being transformed into reenacting the very problem the family needs to address?" The point of staying aware of self-experience is to direct our comments in a way that helps people recognize just those taken-for-granted experiences that relational psychologist Christopher Bollas calls, "the unthought known." This phenomenon is one of the forces that ultimately keep people stuck.

There are several types of transformations that can help child professionals make sense of unexpectedly intense reactions to teens.

OBVIOUS TRANSFORMATIONS

Some transformations are almost impossible to miss. Helen was a supervisee in my training program. During the first session with an overwhelmed mother and her two unruly children, she gave the family *six* homework assignments, *all due the following week.* Helen also reported feeling frazzled in the meeting and unable to pay any attention to what the kids were saying. Here was an obvious transformation! Helen had always been a cool, clear thinker, an excellent listener, and philosophically opposed to being overly directive with families. Believing that this uncharacteristic response might be useful, I asked her to mention during the next meeting that she had been too demanding with the assignments. I also asked her to find out if anyone else in the family made such unrealistic demands.

As it turned out, both Mother and Father were "driven," highly compulsive people—much like Helen during the session. Mother constantly created lists of tasks for Father and the children, and Dad, while ignoring *her* lists, made the lives of his work subordinates miserable with his equally lengthy and elaborate requirements. Both spent so much time directing that they had lost effective control over their children who, feeling overwhelmed, were always on the verge of rebellion.

Helen's transformation into an overwhelming and overwhelmed taskmaster was a critical sign showing her how to engage these parents and kids. Her words to them were simple: "I apologize for giving you so much to do. It felt terrible to me," Helen continued, shaking her head, "to be so frazzled. I now have a feeling what it's like for you."

Another example: A therapist I supervised was extremely judgmental and angry toward Amber, a 15-year-old client. Amber wouldn't let the therapist speak without interrupting. She changed the subject constantly, and made it very clear (when she whistled pop tunes) that she wasn't listening. The therapist was surprised at her own level of irritation over this rude but not outlandish teen behavior. We viewed her reaction as a transformation—a signal that some important issue about Amber and her family had not been addressed, specifically how family conversations went and how Amber made her presence known.

Countertransference reactions can be explored either with the client or by calling a focused family session. Amber's therapist decided to hold a family session. It became clear almost immediately from the interaction that everyone constantly interrupted everyone else. In addition, Amber's parents were subtly judgmental about their daughter's difficulty keeping up. Quite obviously, the therapist's uncharacteristic annoyance was a vivid signal about what needed to be addressed.

Group Supervision Transformations

Transformations also occur in the "parallel process" of group supervision. How the group responds toward a particular case, compared to its usual ethos, is often a signal about what is *not* being addressed in treatment. For example, a counselor at one of our meetings—I had been supervising this group for over a decade and knew the therapists extremely well—reported on his work with Joey, an extremely depressed 16-year-old from a family that had recently immigrated to this country. In an atypical way, the group became incensed, furious at Joey's mother, and vehemently took his side against Mom. The reaction was so negative toward this mom, and so empathic toward Joey, that it was a red flag, impossible to ignore. I said: "You need to get the family in and see what's happening there, because this group never reacts in such a ferociously negative way." The therapist did bring this up with Joey and the family. He quickly realized that everyone—the boy, his father, and both grandmothers—blamed Mom for what they considered her grossly inadequate mothering. Because of her efforts to help Joey assimilate into the larger culture, Mother was being heaped with blame for turning him into "an American," an attack that our group, in its own unconscious wisdom, was registering. Until this harsh but subtle blame was addressed, until Joey 'fessed up to his own fascination with America's pop culture, he wasn't going to get better.

A Slightly Off-Beat Transformation

In one of the more bizarre examples of transformation I've witnessed, a highly experienced therapist, Joan, was seeing a family with several kids, including a 16-year-old boy. This teen stood out. Provocative in his dress—tattoos, black nail polish, tight leather pants, and boots—he seemed to run the session. Despite the presence of several adults and siblings, the therapist felt that this teenager was actually in charge of the meeting. Joan couldn't figure out how to be authoritative in sessions. She felt utterly helpless—almost, she absentmindedly said to the group, as if she were "tied up." This reaction was highly unusual for such a veteran clinician. I said, "Do you know much about what he's doing? Do you know about his life, how he spends his weekends? Or does he have you so tied up that you aren't finding out what's really happening?" I gave her a little encouragement to push, to not feel so overpowered. When Joan did, she learned in a private meeting with him, and unbeknownst to the family, that he led a whole other, after-school life as an S&M escort. This was his world behind the wall of silence, in which he regularly met with consenting men and women and engaged in sadomasochistic fantasy-play. Needless to say, the supervision group was stunned to discover the accuracy of the therapist's uncomfortable reactions.

ACTING-OUT TRANSFORMATIONS

The second kind of obvious response we must heed is not just what we feel, but how we act it out. All counselors are guilty of occasionally inexplicable actions. We feel bad about them because they are in the strictest sense "unprofessional." However, when we pay attention and use these uncharacteristic behaviors as signals, they can guide us in the right direction. Again, this is particularly true when working with adolescents. Since teens act out all the time, our countertransferential behavior can be pretty dramatic, too.

A "Lapse of Memory" Transformation

For example, my client Matthew missed a session, and I totally forgot to call him that afternoon or evening, as I normally would do. I remembered, but put it off for several days—highly unusual for me with teens. Here was a classic example of acting out. Almost invariably, when we veer from our usual practice and don't follow up or check on a client's absence, we are acting out something important the adults are ignoring. In Matthew's case, my not calling was a signal of serious fragmentation in the family. Matthew's mother and father were absent. He had complete freedom to move around town with no one having any idea of his whereabouts. This was no small matter, since his life included compulsive poker playing, plots of revenge against kids who had "wronged" him, and excessive drinking.

A Lack of Curiosity Transformation

One therapist I supervised, Marge, was on such friendly terms with the parents of a girl she was seeing that she abandoned her usual curiosity, rarely probing or asking questions to get beneath the surface. Everything was delightfully casual. Interestingly, Marge also learned little about what was going on from her equally friendly teen client. Everyone was as happy as a clam, but treatment wasn't getting anywhere. With a lot of encouragement, Marge called them in for a family session. The meeting proved just as "feel-good" as all other contacts. Marge finally recognized her unusual easygoing stance and decided to ask for private meetings with each parent. Suddenly, Marge was back to her curious self. And, what surprises there were: Both parents had kept secrets from each other; both were having affairs and both "knew" but didn't know. In addition, their adolescent daughter had her own secret world. She was binge eating and purging. None of this came to the surface until Marge stopped acting out a profound lack of curiosity, helping Mom and Dad stay off the hook. When Marge started to push, these critical issues literally erupted into the work. It was a terrible mess to clean up, and understandable why even this veteran therapist had skated across the smooth surface.

MONEY TRANSFORMATIONS

A key area in which professionals act out family dynamics centers on billing and the finances of treatment. Aside from personal issues about money (which most of us have), acting out in this area is a "transformation" that often has to do with unaddressed family issues regarding finances. In one such case, a counselor was unusually negligent in taking care of bills—no matter how often the supervision group or agency administration reminded him. It almost seemed as if he *refused* to hand over or even mail bills to this family. Finally, after considerable cajoling by his peer supervision group, the therapist started to ask how money was handled in the family. Not surprisingly, it turned out to be *the* central issue that was driving Drew, his 15-year-old client, crazy. Drew's father used money to control. He doled it out according to how "good" each family member was behaving and how well the kids were doing their schoolwork. When the therapist finally billed the family, Dad created a maddeningly slow payment schedule. By now this mild-mannered clinician had become absolutely furious with Dad. Edgar Levenson might well have said, "Told you so!" as the counselor was transformed into an outraged adolescent. He never could confront Dad, a smooth-talking construction-site manager, about his withholding cash. But, Drew had created his own classic teen response. A year later the therapist found out he'd been skimming money from home: stealing small bills from pockets and "borrowing" change in such a stealth way, no one had even noticed.

A "Money Back Guarantee" Transformation

In another case on which I consulted, 14-year-old Anne had been so vicious toward her mom, so unabashedly relentless in her teen contempt and derisive back talk, that the normally firm therapist felt intense guilt toward Mom about being unable to crack this abusive pattern. Here, the therapist, without discussing it in peer supervision, acted out her guilt out by unilaterally reducing the family's sliding scale fee by 50%. Yes, the family was hard-pressed, but this act of benevolence was a Levensonian transformation, a guilt-inspired enactment of the mother's ineffectiveness with her daughter. Once done, it was as if the therapist, along with Mom, had entirely given up. Anne felt the loss of limits and spiraled further and further into the second family. Here was a girl without an envelope at home, who fell ever more deeply into her second family's romance with urban street-life.

SUBTLE TRANSFORMATIONS

Transformational signals occur at the edge of consciousness. By this I mean subtle moods fleeting thoughts, recurring fantasies, songs, and night dreams. Teens get under our skin. Their outlandish behavior, life-and-death decisions, and constant high drama are not lost on one's unconscious. Professionals who work with adolescents should pay special attention to the world just between conscious and unconscious process—subtle experience provides clues that reflect unaddressed dynamics or even about-to-happen events.

A "You're Smarter Than You Think" Transformation

A 15-year-old boy, Ian, who was on the verge of expulsion from his third school, an alternative, urban public school "without walls," was talking with me about his "last chance" term paper project. "Blow this and I'm out," he admitted. I nodded wisely in agreement. At the same time, though, I had a half-second fleeting thought that the term paper might actually be a figment of his imagination. Impossible, I immediately concluded—the details he discussed were all too clear and specific. Sure enough, my unconscious was telling us both something. Weeks later I found out that Ian (like many other 21st-century kids I've worked with), turned in a completely plagiarized paper. He was busted by the school and sent packing once again. My doubt lasted for a nanosecond, almost too fast to register. But that is exactly the nature of such fleeting countertransferential red flags.

A "When Is This Session Finally Going to Be Over?" Transformation

At one point, I was seeing Devin, a 16-year-old client. In our sessions, I found myself unusually bored. There was a palpable flatness to our meetings; they just didn't resonate with the vibrancy you so often feel when working with adolescents. I was going a little stir-crazy, hoping that he'd cancel or forget sessions (many therapists can relate to this). I brought up the issue directly with Devin and said, "I feel more bored with you than I usually feel. Something isn't right here and I want to know what's going on." I finally began to do some detailed digging into his day-to-day behavior, and, reluctantly, Devin revealed that he and a couple of his friends were engaged in huge amounts of daily pot smoking. Devin had flattened himself out so much he diluted the edge of my typical responses to teens in treatment.

Uncanny Unconscious Transformations

Armand was a loner, an outcast in his school, a boy who sullenly roamed through the world of violent cyberspace fantasy games. Post-Columbine, this was a therapist's nightmare, which I literally had several times about Armand—dream sequences of him wreaking havoc in school. Armand never said anything about revenge per se; he was ostensibly antiwar and had no access to guns in his home. But my dreams told a different story. Finally, I brought up my fantasies about his inner world. "Armand, are you telling me what you think about? Do you want to get revenge against those kids who dissed you?" As if on cue, he divulged his astonishingly aggressive inner world, detailed stories of superheroes and villains set out to destroy each other. Though never an actual threat to anyone (except subtly to himself), Armand's hidden experience was one of nonstop aggression and redemption. He admitted envying the "courage of those Columbine kids" (not the first kid to tell me this), but instead lived it all out in his private creations. My dreams revealed something important; they led to many discussions about mastering his rage and the nuances of the social scene, discussions that over time moved him into the real world of relationships. Then, just as I've warned, Armand's newfound "health" put him in harm's way—now he was increasingly exposed to the ordinary adolescent world of binge drinking, smoking, unsafe sex, and second-family feuds.

Dreams are gifts when working with volatile teens who constantly deal with high-risk behaviors. Kids kick up the dust of our own growing-up experiences; they leave a "residue" of emotional signals during sessions. When 14-year-old Wendy came to a meeting with a couple of her girlfriends, they seemed appropriately giggly and affectionate with each other. In my dreams that night however, they were smoking pot for the first time. Sure enough, the next session Wendy casually reported that they'd gone straight from the session and, as secretly planned, had gotten thoroughly "wasted" and almost arrested in the park.

An "I-Tune" Transformation

Working with another teen, a 16-year-old severely withdrawn girl, Constance, I could not get Roberta Flack's song *Killing Me Softly with His Song* out of my head. I worried inordinately about her, despite the fact that Constance was a "model" child. Strangely, though I loved Roberta Flack's song, I had not heard it in years. I passed it off as just another bit of mental debris—until this heretofore soft-spoken girl erupted in a fit of near-psychotic rage that shocked all around, including me. A thorough psychiatric evaluation uncovered a bipolar disorder that required mood-stabilizing medication. Constance's quiet demeanor belied her fast-cycling mood swings and history of rage attacks directed against family members. Constance had begun to take me into her orbit and I was, as my unconscious tried to warn me, a potential object of her rage.

Obvious transformations, acting-out transformations, financial transformations, and subtle transformations. For any professional working with adolescents, these "unprofessional" experiences are a gift. If we maintain an internal dialogue with ourselves ("Is this response characteristic of me or is it unusual?"), they can be signals.

They help us understand the unspoken; they allow us to see behind the wall of silence, and move kids toward healthier decisions.

Afterword

This "real-in-relational" challenge of working with teens is a fitting place to end. It is a perfect metaphor for adolescence: we must try not to be ashamed of the different kinds of experiences we have. Outrageous teen behavior is a stark message to us that we must continue to grow along with them. Being provocateurs at heart, wanting the best for the vulnerable adults who must guide them, adolescents offer us maddening challenges and an ultimate joy.

♦ Kids challenge us to recognize how their world is truly changing—almost faster than we can keep up with it.

♦ Teens challenge us to stay professionally open minded, to integrate our views rather than promote narrow "cliques" with all or none approaches.

♦ Adolescents challenge us to stretch ourselves and—like the second family—to share with each other what works and what does not work.

In the end, then, it is not just about the kids. It is about us as people, parents, and child professionals. Ultimately, it is the challenge and joy of realizing that it is never too late to change.

BIBLIOGRAPHY

Bakeman, Roger, & Gottman, John M. (1997). *Observing interaction: An introduction to sequential analysis.* New York: Cambridge University Press.

Balint, Michael. (1968). *The basic fault.* Evanston, IL: Northwestern University Press.

Bennett, William. (1993).*The book of virtues.* New York: Simon & Schuster.

Bollas, Christopher. (1987). *The shadow of the object.* New York: Columbia University Press.

Deci, Edward L. (1995). *Why we do what we do.* New York: Penguin Books.

Denizet-Lewis, Benoit. (2004, May 30). Friends, friends with benefits and the benefits of the local mall. *The New York Times,* Section 6, p. 30.

Ehrenberg, Darlene. (1992). *The intimate edge: Extending the reach of psychoanalytic interaction.* New York: Norton.

Emerson, Judy. (1996, December 20). Hearing our future. *Rockford Register Star.* Rockford, IL.

Eyre, Linda, & Eyre, Richard. (1993). *Teaching children values.* New York: Simon & Schuster.

Ginott, Haim G. (1965). *Between parent and child.* New York: Macmillan.

Gordon, Thomas. (1970). *Parent effectiveness training.* New York: P.H. Wyden.

Gosman, Fred G. (1990). *Spoiled rotten.* New York: Villard.

Grunbaum, J., Kann, L., Kinchen, S., et al. (2003). *2003 youth high risk behavior survey.* Centers for Disease Control and Prevention, Department of Health and Human Services, Atlanta Georgia.

Hoffman, Irwin Z. (1998). The patient as interpreter of the analyst's experience. In *Ritual and spontaneity in the psychoanalytic process.* Hillside, NJ: Analytic Press.

Klein, Melanie. (1949). *The psychoanalysis of children.* London: Hogarth Press.

Kohut, Heinz. (1971). *The analysis of the self* (Psychoanalysis of the Child Monograph No. 4). Madison, CT: International Universities Press.

Laing, R. D. (1969). *The divided self.* London: Penguin.

Lerner, Barbara. (1972). *Therapy in the ghetto: Political impotence and personal integration.* Baltimore: Johns Hopkins University Press.

Lerner, Harriet. (1985). *The dance of anger.* New York: Harper & Row.

Levenson, Edgar A. (1972). *The fallacy of understanding.* New York: Basic Books.

Levine, Melvin D. (2002). *A mind at a time.* New York: Simon & Schuster.

Mahler, Margaret, Pine, Fred, & Bergman, Anni. (1975). *The psychological birth of the human infant.* New York: Basic Books.

Miller, Alice. (1981). *Prisoners of childhood.* New York: Basic Books.

Roberts, D. F., Foehr, U. G., Rideout, V. J., & Brodie, M. (1999, November). *Kids and media at the new millennium* (*A Kaiser Family Foundation Report*). Menlo Park, CA: Kaiser Family Foundation.

Roth, Phillip. (1969). *Portnoy's complaint.* New York: Random House.

Seligman, Martin E. (1995). *The optimistic child.* Boston, MA: Houghton Mifflin.

Shure, Myrna B., with DiGeronimo, Theresa F. (1994). *Raising a thinking child.* New York: Henry Holt.

Simmons, Rachel. (2002). *Odd girl out.* New York: Harcourt.

Stern, Daniel N. (1985). *The interpersonal world of the infant.* New York: Basic Books.

Strupp, Hans. (1977). *Psychotherapy for better or worse.* New York: Aronson.

Taffel, Ron. (2001). *The second family.* New York: St. Martin's Press.

Taffel, Ron. (2001). *Getting through to difficult kids and parents.* New York: Guilford Press.

Taffel, Ron. (1999). *Nurturing good children now.* New York: Golden Books.

Taffel, Ron. (1990, September/October). The politics of mood. *Family Therapy Networker, 14*(5), 49–72.

Taffel, Ron. (1986, November/December). Revolution/evolution: Feminism forces us to reconsider our expectations about dramatic cures. *Family Therapy Networker, 10*(6), 52–58.

Taffel, Ron. (1995, November/December). Honoring the everyday. *Family Therapy Networker, 19*(6), 25–28, 56.

Thurow, Lester C. (1997, January 28). Changes in capitalism render one-earner families obsolete. *USA Today,* p. 7a.

Trebay, Guy. (2003, September 2). The skin wars start earlier and earlier. *The New York Times,* Section B, p. 8.

Winnicott, D. W. (1975). *Through paediatrics to psycho-analysis.* London: Hogarth Press.

INDEX

Abuse
    childrearing techniques as a result of,
        17–18
    of parents by teens, 202–206
Acting-out transformations, 275–276. *See
    also* Transformations
Action-oriented questions, 196
Actions in communication, 264–266
Advice
    compared to being controlling, 120–
        123
    compared to the parent–child
        relationship, 123–125
    details and, 115–120
    importance of, 109–111
    learning styles and, 111–115
    overview, 107–109
    teaching parents to give, 199–202
    unheard, 125–126
Alcohol use
    inquiring about during initial
        sessions, 38–39
    in today's youth culture, 8–10
Anger
    parental, 205
    in today's youth culture, 12–15
Anxiety
    in parenting, 15–17
    in today's youth culture, 10–12
Arguing
    as a learning style, 112–113
    as a passion, 102–104
Assumptions regarding treatment, 28–29
Authority, adult, 14–15

Behavior, controlling
    compared to giving advice, 120–123
    tough love parenting and, 179

Behavioral change
    in focused family sessions, 216–218
    moving towards, 226–227
    sense of self and, 4
    therapeutic relationship and, 27–28
    transformations as, 270–280
Body language, 264–266
Boredom
    three-dimensional therapist and, 262–
        263
    as a transformation, 278–279
Brain functioning, 25–26

Celebrity culture, 19–20. *See also* Pop
    culture
Challenging kids
    divided self and, 75
    to empathize with parents, 82–92
    in focused family sessions, 228–231
    overview, 73–74, 75–76
    to talk to their parents more, 76–82
Challenging ourselves, 259–260
Challenging parents, 231–232
Change. *See also* Transformations
    in focused family sessions, 216–218
    moving towards, 226–227
    sense of self and, 4
    therapeutic relationship and, 27–28
Childrearing. *See also* Parent–child
        relationship; Parents
    advice and, 199–202
    confidentiality in treatment and, 149
    conflict discussions and, 197–199
    confusion regarding, 15–17, 181
    consequences and, 185–188
    creating a home teens love and, 209–
        211
    divided self and, 74–75